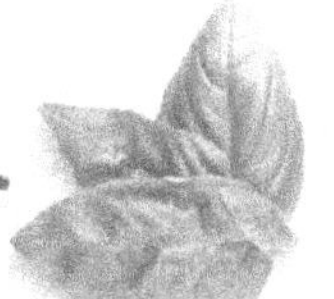

Complete FATTY LIVER DIET COOKBOOK FOR SENIORS

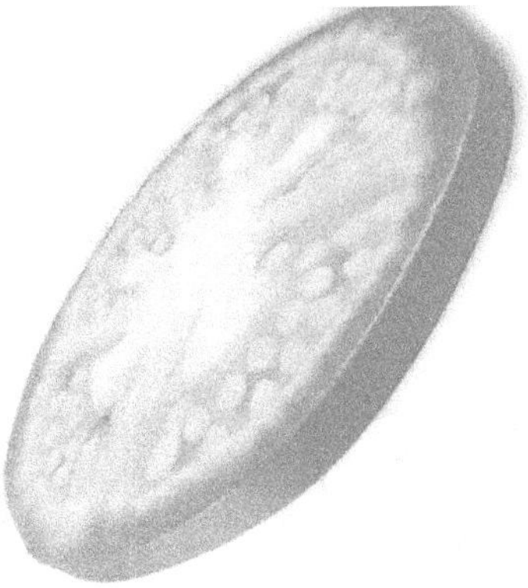

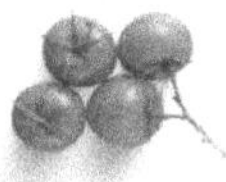

Boost Your Vitality and Purify Your Body with Easy and Delicious Recipes. Comes with a 60-Day Meal Plan and a Useful Bonus

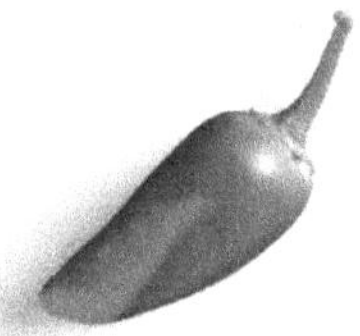

Sarah William

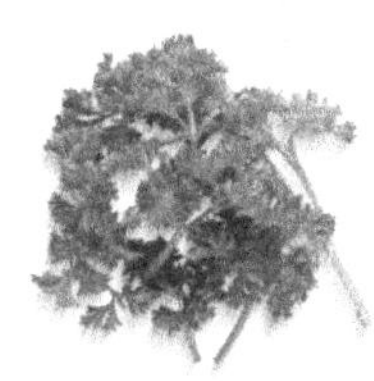

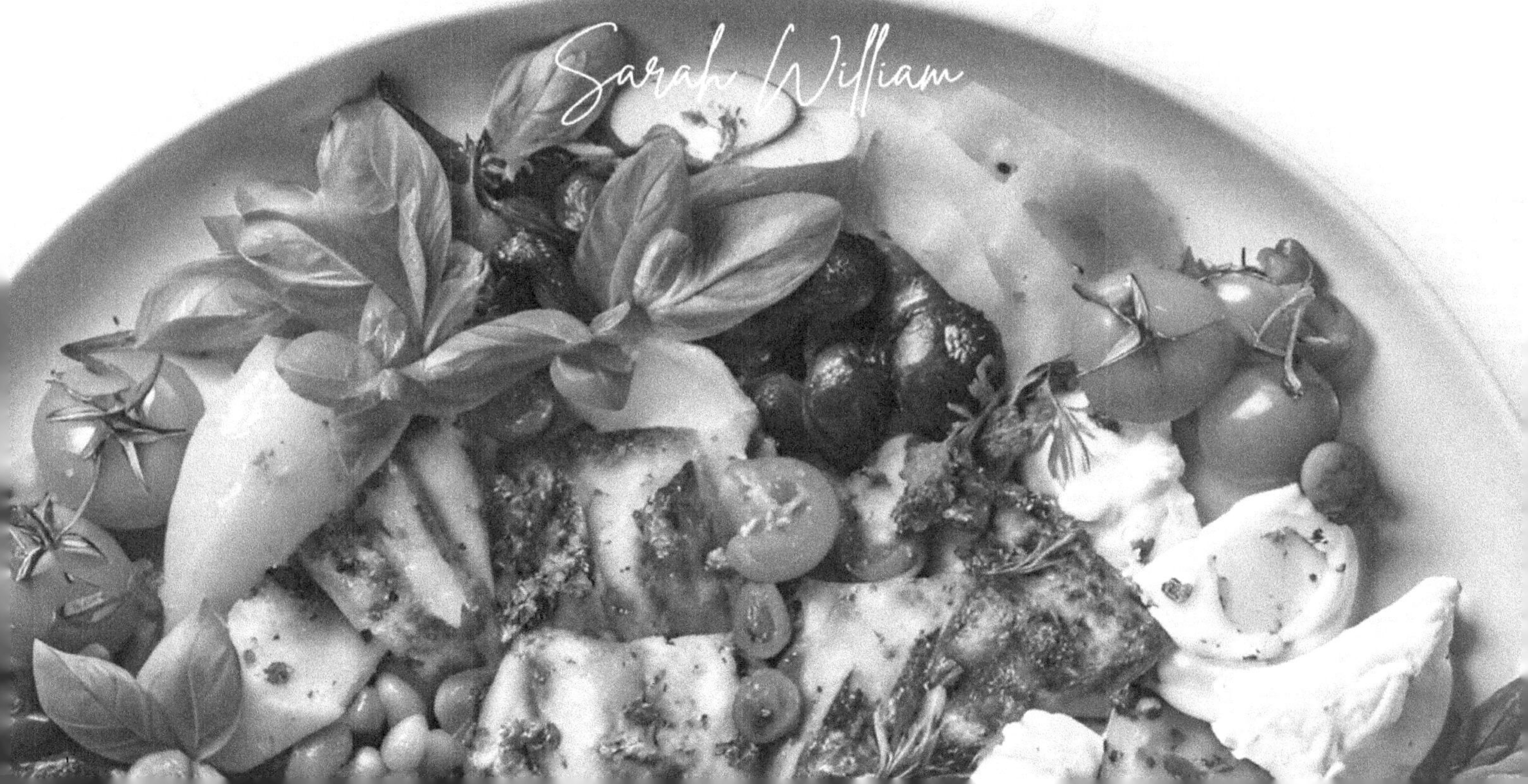

Table of Contents

Dedication

To all those who strive for a healthier tomorrow, May this book serve as a guiding light on your journey to wellness.

BONUS AWAIT YOU !
SCAN THE QR CODE
BELOW

THANK YOU!

Introduction

Imagine yourself in your doctor's office, hearing the devastating news that you have fatty liver disease. All of a sudden, you feel a surge of shock and disorientation. What is meant by this? What caused it to occur? What's more, what can you do about it?

I'm here to inform you that you're not alone. Millions of individuals worldwide suffer from fatty liver disease, which is more widespread than you may imagine. The shocking thing is that your liver isn't the only factor. Studies reveal a wide range of health problems, including diabetes, obesity, heart disease, and potentially cancer, are associated with fatty liver disease. Sounds scary?

From this point on, things become fascinating. Fatty liver disease doesn't have to be a death sentence, even if it often seems like one. Yes, hope still exists! It all starts with the food you put on your plate.

As a nutritionist, I've dug deep into the field of fatty liver disease, reading through a ton of literature to find the keys to curing this problem. And believe me, you will be shocked by what I discovered.

Were you aware that little dietary adjustments might have a significant effect on liver health? It is accurate! You may not only stop the growth of fatty liver disease but also reverse it by giving up processed junk food and eating an abundance of nutrient-rich meals. Yes, you did hear me correctly. Turn it wrong.

Here's the thing, though: I understand. Changing a diet might be intimidating, particularly if you're used to a certain eating style. That's what this book does.

These pages contain a wealth of delectable dishes designed to satisfy your appetite and tantalize your taste buds. Every meal is made with love and supported by research, ranging from filling breakfasts to delicious dinners and everything in between.

Still, that's not all. To eliminate confusion around mealtimes, I have also created a 60-day eating plan. You'll have everything you need to get started on improved liver health, including thorough shopping lists and simple-to-follow recipes.
What, then, do you say? Are you prepared to take charge of your health and make a radical internal change in your life? Then grab a seat; this book will take you on an adventure of a lifetime.
Prepare to be shocked—in the greatest possible way—by your liver. Let's get started!"

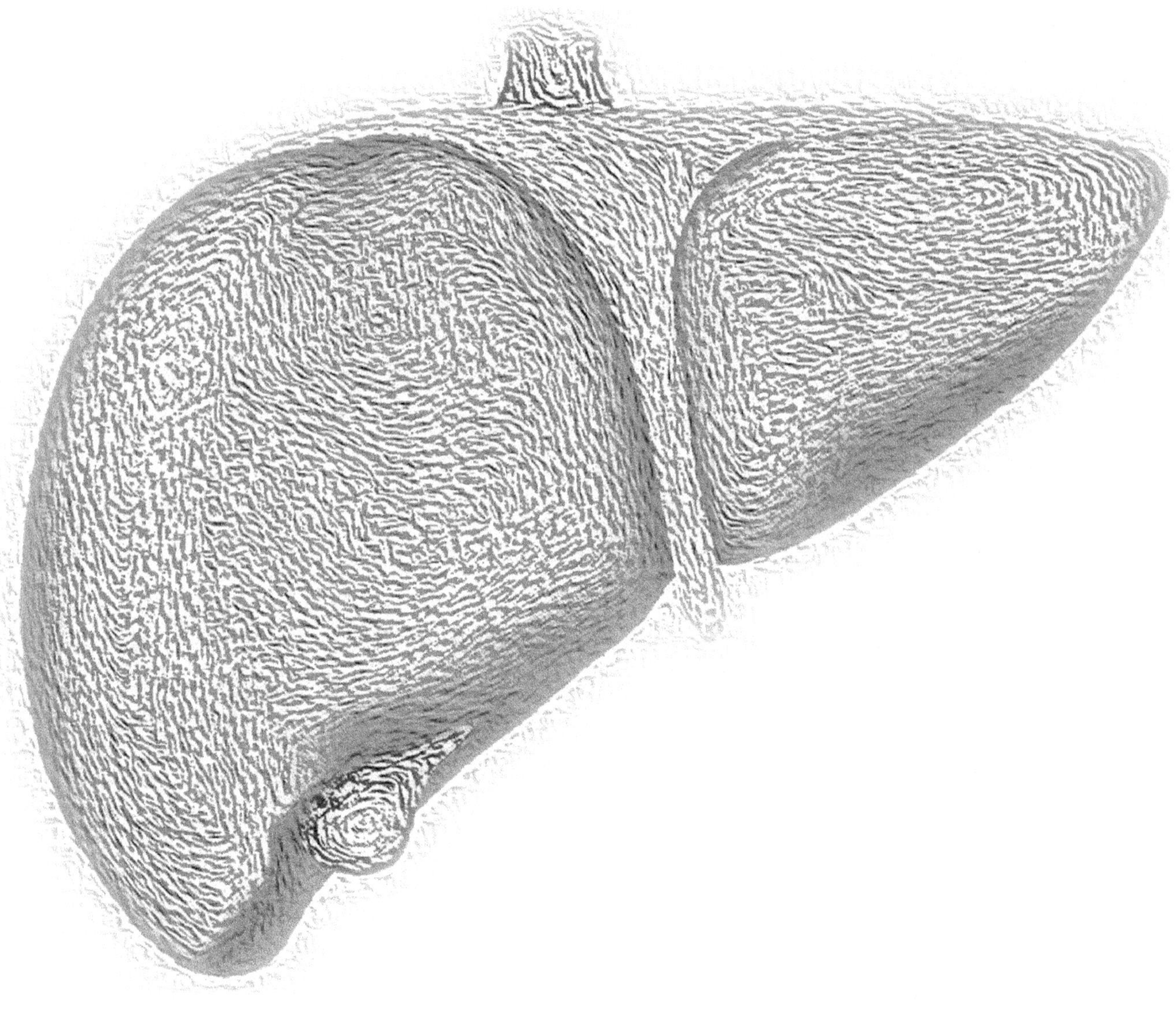

Welcome Message

Hello and welcome to the "Fatty Liver Cookbook for Seniors: Boost Your Vitality and Purify Your Body with Easy and Delicious Recipes." It is a great pleasure for me to welcome you to the book. Let me begin by telling you a personal experience that inspired it.

My mother was identified as having fatty liver disease a few years ago. As a nutritionist, I was aware of the importance of food and lifestyle in controlling this illness, but going through my mom's journey personally opened my eyes to a new depth of comprehension and empathy. It was difficult to see her battle with exhaustion, pain, and anxiety about the possible implications of this diagnosis for her future. However, it also stoked my desire to utilize my knowledge and abilities to change the world.

She stated, "I want to get better, but I don't know where to start," as we sat at the kitchen table one evening. She had a worried expression on her face. For us both, it was a turning point. I realized that while the knowledge was there, it needed to be understandable and useful for those like my mother, who wanted to reclaim their health but felt overburdened by the adjustments they had to make.

We set off on a voyage of exploration and metamorphosis together. We looked at dishes that were tasty, simple to make, and packed with nutrients. We created flexible but organized meal plans so she could enjoy eating without feeling cheated. Most significantly, we discovered how to maintain these modifications, making healthy eating a way of life rather than a band-aid solution.

This cookbook is the result of that journey. It is crammed with meal plans, recipes, and advice that not only helped my mother manage her fatty liver disease but also allowed her to have a vibrant, active life. Every formulation has undergone extensive testing and refinement to guarantee that it is palatable and healthy for the liver. The bonus section includes further advice on keeping your liver healthy, and the 60-day food plan offers thorough guidance to help you get started and remain on track.

I hope that this book will be a useful tool for you and your family, offering the direction and motivation required to enhance liver function and general health. This cookbook provides useful, tasty, and efficient solutions, whether you're just starting or want to improve your present strategy.

I appreciate being able to share in your adventure. Together, let's go on the journey to improved health.

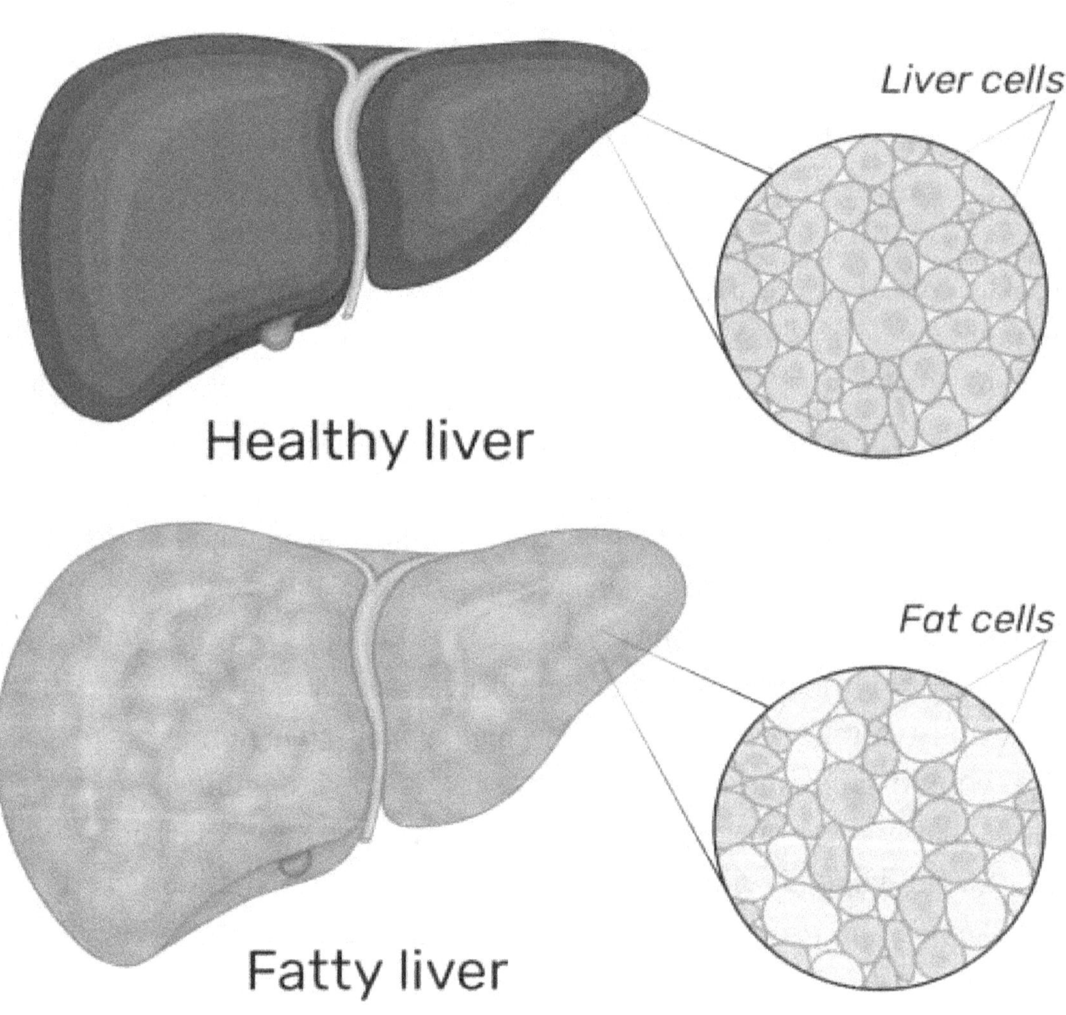

Understanding Fatty Liver Disease

What is Fatty Liver Disease?

Well, let's dissect it now. Have you heard of fatty liver disease before? Otherwise, be ready for a crash lesson on what can be hiding in your liver.

So, let me explain. Like your body's MVP, your liver works tirelessly to maintain proper function. But sometimes, particularly when you throw too much crap at it, it becomes a bit overwhelming.

We then develop fatty liver disease. Imagine if your liver begins to store fat in its cells as a squirrel does, burying them there for the winter, as if calories were a fad. The difficulty starts when fat overwhelms your liver. This may happen quickly.

This is when it starts to get interesting. Oh no, fatty liver disease is more than just some extra padding around your liver that doesn't hurt. It is an indicator that something is wrong with your body—a warning flag.

According to research, fatty liver disease is more than just a cosmetic concern; it's a ticking time bomb that might blow up into a whole other set of health issues. We are discussing liver failure, heart disease, and diabetes. Indeed, frightening stuff.

The worst part is that fatty liver disease is universal. Regardless of age, gender, or lifestyle, everyone may experience it. Your liver may be quietly drowning behind a covering of fat, even if you appear to be in perfect condition on the inside.

As a result, what can you do? And that's what this book does. We'll go into the realm of fatty liver disease and discover the keys to curing it, so you can get your health back.

Prepare to welcome a happier, healthier self and bid fatty liver disease a fond farewell. It's time to reclaim your life and your liver.

Types: NAFLD vs. AFLD

All right, let's speak about kinds. There isn't a one-size-fits-all approach to fatty liver disease. Nope, NAFLD and AFLD are the two primary participants in this game. What then makes a difference? Fasten your seatbelts, as we are about to discover.

First up, for those keeping score at home, we have non-alcoholic fatty liver disease, or NAFLD. Now, despite what the name implies, excessive bottle banging isn't the cause of this particular kind of fatty liver disease. Rather, lifestyle variables such as heredity, food, and exercise—or lack thereof—are often associated with it.

When it comes to liver problems, NAFLD is like the silent killer—sly, nuanced, and all too frequent. Since NAFLD is thought to affect up to 25% of the global population, it is a serious public health problem. The worst part is that most individuals are unaware of their condition until it is too late.

But don't worry—our goal isn't to terrify you. We are here to provide you with the information and resources you need to retaliate against NAFLD. You should not underestimate this opponent, I assure you.

Let's move on to AFLD, sometimes referred to as alcoholic fatty liver disease. This kind of fatty liver disease, unlike NAFLD, is directly related to overindulging in alcohol. Yes, everything I said about your nightly glass of wine or weekend bender may not be as healthy as you think.

The liver's way of suggesting, "Hey, maybe ease up on the booze, huh?" is similar to AFLD. It's an indicator that your liver is having trouble processing the alcohol you consume, and if you ignore it, things might quickly become worse.

The good news is that there is still hope if you have either AFLD, NAFLD, or both. You can recover your liver and your life by treating fatty liver disease with the correct diet, lifestyle modifications, and TLC.

Symptoms and Risk Factors

All right, let's get straight to the point: risk factors and symptoms. Since awareness of potential risk factors and warning signs is half the fight against fatty liver disease, Let's now explore and find out what signals your body may be sending you.

Symptoms come first. This is where things get tricky: fatty liver disease may strike out of the blue like a ninja. You may not even have been aware of a problem in the beginning. However, as the illness worsens, your liver will begin to make loud and unmistakable distress calls.

Imagine persistent exhaustion, pain, or discomfort in your upper right abdomen or inexplicable weight loss. All of them are warning signs that there is a problem with your liver section.

The worst part is that fatty liver disease cannot be diagnosed based just on symptoms. Nope, to get to the bottom of things, you'll have to dig a little bit deeper and roll up your sleeves.

Let's talk about the risk factors. These bad guys are the equivalent of the breadcrumbs that lead directly to the guilty party. And there are enough of them to go around, I promise.

Let's speak about lifestyle first. You may be inviting trouble if your concept of a balanced diet consists more of fries and burgers than fruits and vegetables. Similar to going through the drive-through rather than the gym.

We'll talk about health conditions next. Consider obesity, diabetes, and high cholesterol; these conditions may all get along with fatty liver disease like old friends at a reunion.

Genetics should not be overlooked. You may be more susceptible to fatty liver disease than a normal person.

The truth, however, is that having a few risk factors does not guarantee that you will always have liver problems. Nope, it just indicates that you have a warning and an opportunity to act before things get out of hand.

Now, what say you? Are you prepared to hear what your body is attempting to tell you? Are you prepared to take control of your health and eliminate fatty liver disease? I believed that. Let's get started and discover everything there is to know about risk factors and symptoms. Regaining control over your liver and your life is what's needed.

Importance of Diet and Lifestyle

Effectively treating fatty liver disease requires an understanding of the critical roles that nutrition and lifestyle play in enhancing liver health and general well-being. Let's examine why it's so crucial to make good decisions in these areas:

1. Nutrition:

A diet high in nutrients is essential for maintaining liver health and preventing fatty liver disease. This is the reason why:

Nutrient Density: Eating a diet high in antioxidants, vitamins, and minerals supports the health of the liver and lowers inflammation. Your meals should be built around nutritious grains, lean meats, fresh produce, and healthy fats.

Balanced Macronutrients: Sustaining liver function, controlling blood sugar, and sustaining energy levels all depend on consuming the right amounts of lipids, proteins, and carbs. To encourage satiety and regulate blood sugar levels, concentrate on including complex carbs, lean proteins, and healthy fats in your meals.

Fiber Intake: Consuming enough fiber helps the body rid itself of impurities and maintain digestive health. Consume a diet rich in fruits, vegetables, legumes, whole grains, and other fiber-rich foods to aid in the process of liver detoxification.

Reducing Sugar and Processed Food Consumption: Consuming sugar and processed foods in excess may lead to inflammation and the buildup of liver fat. Eat fewer processed snacks, sugar-filled drinks, and refined carbs to lessen the strain on your liver.

2. Way of Life:

Apart from dietary variables, lifestyle factors are crucial in the management of fatty liver disease.

Frequent Exercise: Regular exercise promotes weight reduction, lowers the buildup of liver fat, and improves insulin sensitivity. To support liver health, try to get in at least 30 minutes of moderate-intensity activity most days of the week.

Retaining a Healthy Weight: To reduce liver fat and improve general health, one must achieve and maintain a healthy weight. You may boost liver function and lose weight by implementing a regular physical exercise routine and eating a balanced diet.

Reducing or Quitting Alcohol: For those with alcoholic fatty liver disease, reducing or quitting alcohol is critical to stop more liver damage. If you drink alcohol often, moderation is essential to maintaining the health of your liver.

Handling Stress: Prolonged stress has been linked to liver damage and inflammation. To promote general well-being, include stress-relieving practices into your daily routine, such as mindfulness, meditation, yoga, or hobbies.

You may actively manage fatty liver disease and promote optimum liver health by making a nutrient-rich diet a priority and leading a healthy lifestyle. Recall that little adjustments may have a significant impact on your liver's health and general well-being.

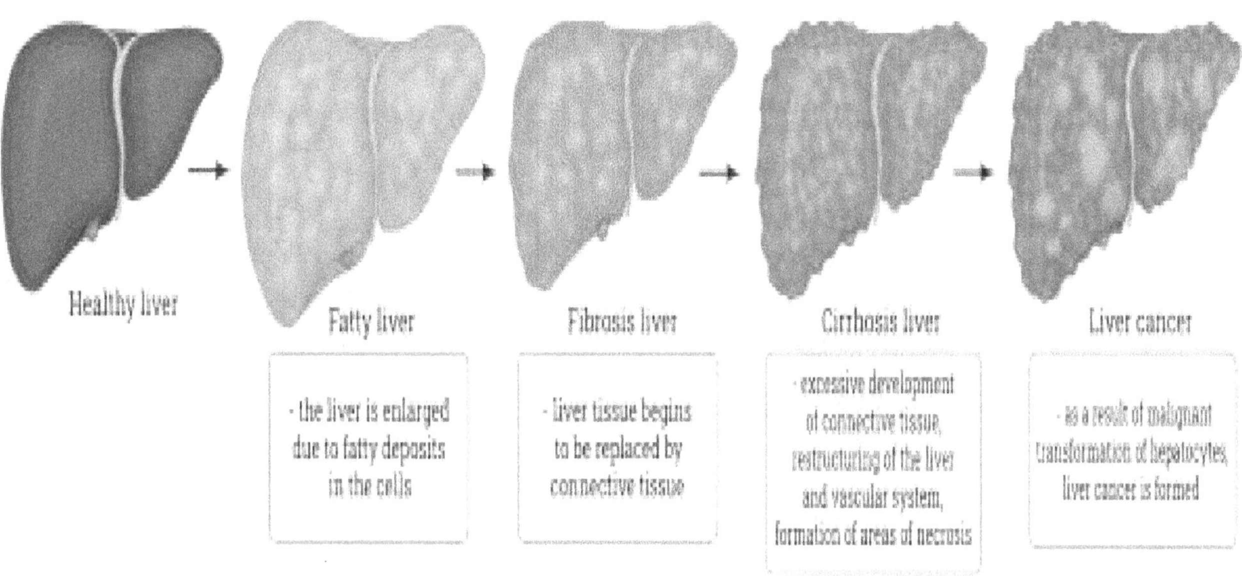

Chapter 1: Getting Started
Basics of a Liver-Friendly Diet

Key Nutrients and Foods to Include

Optimizing your diet with key nutrients and wholesome foods is fundamental to supporting liver health and combating fatty liver disease. Let's explore the essential nutrients and the foods that are rich sources of them:

1. Omega-3 Fatty Acids:

Omega-3 fatty acids are renowned for their anti-inflammatory properties, making them invaluable for reducing liver inflammation and promoting overall liver health. Incorporate sources of omega-3s into your diet, such as:

- Fatty fish: salmon, mackerel, sardines, and trout
- Flaxseeds and chia seeds
- Walnuts
- Hemp seeds

2. Antioxidants:

Antioxidants help neutralize harmful free radicals and protect liver cells from damage. Aim to include a variety of antioxidant-rich foods in your diet, such as:

- Colorful fruits: berries, oranges, grapes, and kiwi
- Vibrant vegetables: spinach, kale, broccoli, bell peppers, and sweet potatoes
- Herbs and spices: turmeric, cinnamon, ginger, and garlic
- Nuts and seeds: almonds, sunflower seeds, and pumpkin seeds

3. Fiber:

Dietary fiber plays a crucial role in promoting digestion, regulating blood sugar levels, and supporting liver detoxification. Focus on incorporating high-fiber foods into your meals, including:

- Whole grains: oats, quinoa, brown rice, and barley
- Legumes: lentils, chickpeas, black beans, and kidney beans
- Fruits: apples, pears, bananas, and berries
- Vegetables: Brussels sprouts, broccoli, carrots, and artichokes

4. Lean proteins:

Opt for lean protein sources that provide essential amino acids without excess saturated fats, which can contribute to liver inflammation. Include the following protein-rich foods in your diet:

- Poultry: chicken breast and turkey.

- Fish: cod, tilapia, haddock, and halibut
- Plant-based proteins: tofu, tempeh, edamame, and legumes

5. Healthy fats:

Incorporate healthy fat sources that support liver health and provide essential fatty acids. Choose foods rich in monounsaturated and polyunsaturated fats, such as:

- Avocados
- Olive oil
- Nuts and seeds
- Fatty fish

6. Vitamin E:

Vitamin E is an essential antioxidant that helps protect liver cells from damage and inflammation. Include foods rich in vitamin E, such as:

- Almonds
- Sunflower seeds
- Spinach
- Swiss chard
- Avocado

By prioritizing these key nutrients and incorporating a variety of wholesome foods into your diet, you can provide essential support for your liver health and effectively manage fatty liver disease. Remember to focus on a balanced and varied diet to ensure you're meeting all your nutritional needs.

Foods to Avoid

While incorporating nutrient-rich foods into your diet is essential for supporting liver health, it's equally important to minimize or avoid certain foods that can exacerbate fatty liver disease and contribute to liver inflammation. Let's explore the foods you should steer clear of:

1. Sugary foods and beverages:
- **Added Sugars:** Avoid foods and beverages with added sugars, such as sodas, energy drinks, sweetened juices, candies, and baked goods. Excessive sugar consumption can contribute to liver fat accumulation and insulin resistance.

2. Processed and fried foods:
- **Trans Fats:** Limit or avoid foods high in trans fats, including fried foods, processed snacks, baked goods, and margarine. Trans fats promote inflammation and can worsen liver health.

3. High-Sodium Foods:
- **Processed and Packaged Foods:** Reduce your intake of processed and packaged foods, such as canned soups, salty snacks, deli meats, and convenience meals. These foods are often high in sodium, which can contribute to fluid retention and liver damage.

4. Alcohol:
- **Excessive Alcohol Consumption:** If you have alcoholic fatty liver disease or are at risk of developing it, it's crucial to limit or eliminate alcohol consumption altogether. Alcohol is a major contributor to liver inflammation and can exacerbate liver damage.

5. Refined carbohydrates:
- **White Bread, Pasta, and Rice:** Choose whole grain alternatives over refined carbohydrates to support stable blood sugar levels and reduce liver fat accumulation.

6. Saturated and trans fats:

- **Fatty Meats:** Limit your intake of fatty cuts of meat, such as red meat, bacon, sausage, and processed meats. Opt for lean protein sources to reduce saturated fat intake and support liver health.

7. High-Glycemic Index Foods:

- **White Potatoes and White Rice:** Choose low-glycemic index alternatives, such as sweet potatoes, quinoa, and brown rice, to help regulate blood sugar levels and reduce the risk of insulin resistance.

8. Excessive Salt:

- **Table Salt and High-Sodium Condiments:** Limit your use of table salt and high-sodium condiments like soy sauce, ketchup, and salad dressings. Opt for herbs, spices, and vinegar-based dressings to flavor your meals instead.

By minimizing or avoiding these foods and focusing on a diet rich in whole, nutrient-dense foods, you can support liver health, reduce inflammation, and effectively manage fatty liver disease. Remember to read food labels carefully and make mindful choices to prioritize your liver health.

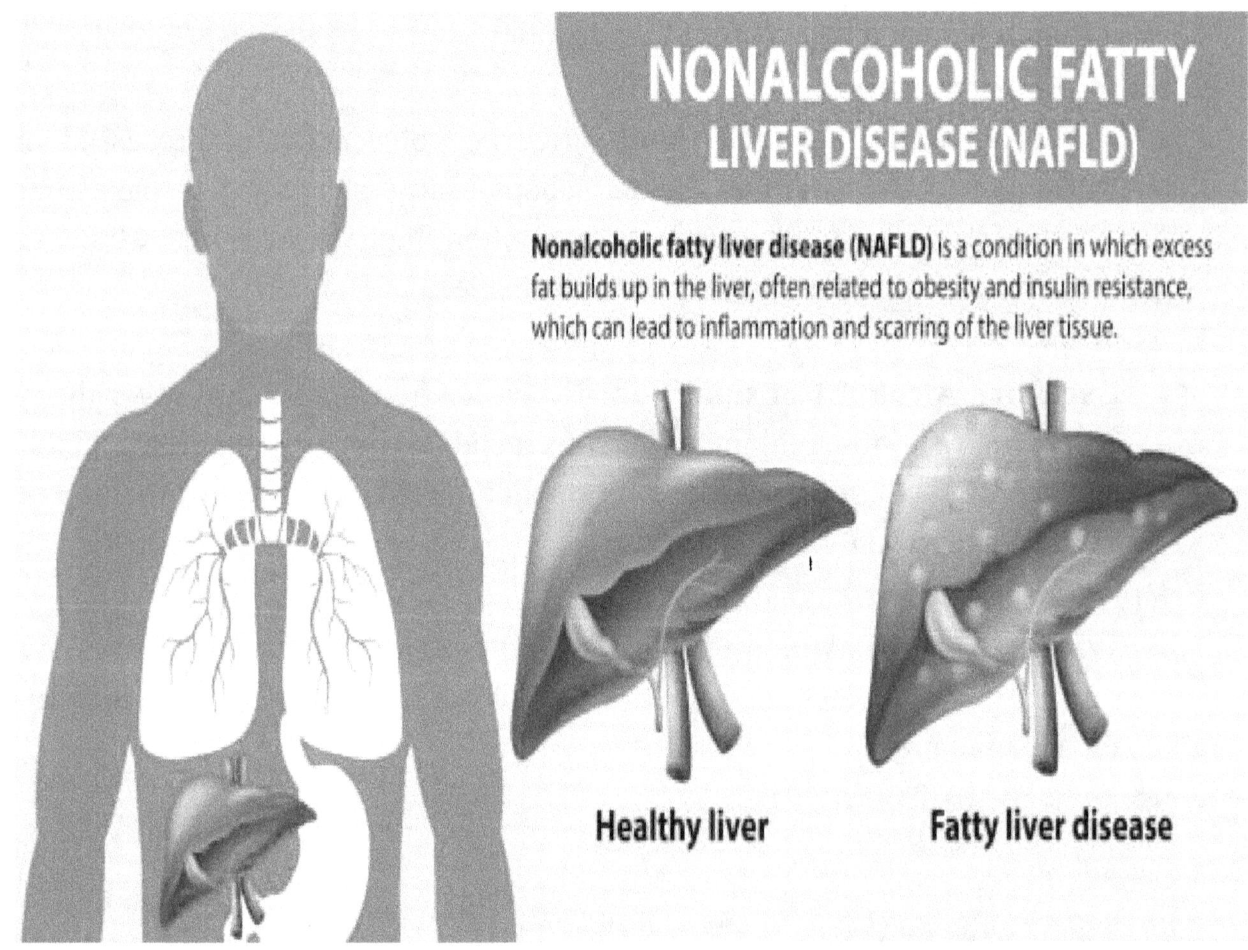

Adapting Recipes for Senior Dietary Needs

Our nutritional requirements may vary as we get older, necessitating dietary adjustments to maintain general health and wellbeing. Seniors with fatty liver disease may benefit from specialized dietary adjustments made to meet their requirements. Here's how to modify dishes to suit the nutritional requirements of seniors:

1. Reduction of Sodium:

Limiting salt consumption may be necessary for seniors to maintain heart health and control diseases like high blood pressure. When modifying recipes to improve taste without sacrificing flavor, consider cutting down on or eliminating added salt and substituting other flavor enhancers like herbs, spices, and citrus zest.

2. Improvement of Fiber:

Consuming enough fiber is critical for maintaining digestive health, blood sugar regulation, and satiety. To increase the amount of fiber in dishes, use high-fiber components such as whole grains, legumes, fruits, and vegetables. Pick dishes that include plenty of vibrant fruits and vegetables along with healthy grains like quinoa, brown rice, and whole wheat pasta.

3. Moderation of Proteins:

Even though protein is necessary to maintain general health and muscle mass, seniors may need to limit their protein consumption, particularly if they have kidney-related issues. Select lean protein sources and use them in dishes in the right amounts, such as fish, chicken, tofu, and lentils.

4. Modification of Texture:

Certain food textures may be challenging for some elderly people to chew or swallow. To make items simpler to eat while changing recipes, think about pureeing, chopping, or mashing them. It is possible to smooth out the textures of soups, stews, and casseroles by blending or straining them, making it easier for elderly people who have trouble swallowing.

5. Control of Portion:

Portion management is crucial to preventing overeating and maintaining a healthy weight when the metabolism slows down with age. When preparing meals, consider using smaller dishes to help reduce quantities, and be mindful of portion proportions. Encourage elders to pay attention to their bodies' signals of hunger and fullness to prevent overindulging.

6. Density of Nutrients:

To promote general health, make sure that meals are nutrient-dense and include vital vitamins, minerals, and antioxidants. To optimize nutritional consumption, include a range of vibrant fruits, veggies, whole grains, lean meats, and healthy fats in your dishes. Select recipes that employ as many whole, unprocessed foods as possible and have an emphasis on nutrient-rich components.

Seniors with special dietary requirements may have tasty and fulfilling meals while receiving enough nutrients if you modify recipes to suit their needs. For individualized nutritional advice based on your health requirements and preferences, think about speaking with a certified dietitian or other healthcare provider.

Easy Cooking Techniques and Kitchen Safety

For elders, cooking should be a fulfilling and joyful experience, but it's critical to put safety and ease of use first in the kitchen. To guarantee a pleasurable cooking experience, consider the following simple cooking methods and safety advice:

1. Make recipes simpler:

Choose recipes that are simple to follow and require only a few materials and processes. Seek out recipes like one-pot meals, sheet pan dinners, and slow cooker dishes that require little preparation time and straightforward cooking methods. As a result, senior citizens will find cooking less intimidating and more pleasurable.

2. Getting the ingredients ready:

In the kitchen, preparing materials in advance may save time and work. To speed up the cooking process, remind elders to wash, cut, and portion their items before cooking. Additionally, preparing ingredients ahead of time might help you follow recipes more easily and stress-free at the last minute.

3. Make Use of Kitchen Utensils:

Seniors cooking may be safer and simpler with the help of kitchen gadgets and appliances. Invest in easy-to-use kitchen gear, including vegetable peelers, chopping boards, sharp knives, and ergonomic kitchenware. Food processors, blenders, and slow cookers are examples of electric gadgets that help streamline culinary chores and lower the possibility of mishaps.

4. Adhere to kitchen safety procedures.

In the kitchen, safety should always come first, particularly for elderly people. Remind elderly people to use appliances, hot surfaces, and sharp items with care. Urge children to handle hot cookware with oven gloves or potholders and to always have a fire extinguisher available for unexpected situations.

5. Keep the kitchen tidy:

Food safety and hygiene depend on a well-organized and clean kitchen. Seniors should be reminded to often clean surfaces, utensils, and appliances to avoid cross-contamination, as well as to wash their hands completely before and after handling food. Remember to check expiration dates and store perishables properly in the refrigerator to ensure food safety.

6. Modify recipes to reduce risk:

When preparing meals for seniors, consider modifying recipes to suit their nutritional needs and food sensitivities. Instead of frying, go for recipes that call for healthier cooking techniques like baking, grilling, steaming, or sautéing. Steer clear of recipes calling for a lot of sugar, salt, or oil, and if feasible, use healthier substitutes.

Seniors may enjoy preparing tasty and healthy meals while lowering the risk of accidents or injury by using these simple cooking methods and kitchen safety precautions. To make mealtimes interesting and pleasurable, seniors should be encouraged to try out different dishes and cooking methods.

Chapter 2: 60-Day Meal Plan

Overview of the Meal Plan

How to Use the Meal Plan

Welcome to your 60-day meal plan designed to support liver health and overall well-being. This guide will help you understand how to effectively use the meal plan to maximize its benefits.

Understanding the Structure

1. **Daily Breakdown:** Each day includes a breakfast, lunch, dinner, snack, and smoothie or drink.
2. **Variety and Balance:** The plan offers a variety of nutrient-dense meals, ensuring a balance of proteins, carbohydrates, fats, vitamins, and minerals.

Customizing Your Plan

1. **Personal Preferences:** Feel free to swap recipes within the same meal category (e.g., breakfast for breakfast) based on your preferences.
2. **Portion Sizes:** Adjust portion sizes according to your nutritional needs, appetite, and dietary goals.
3. **Dietary Restrictions:** Modify recipes to accommodate any allergies, intolerances, or specific dietary requirements.

Preparing Ahead

1. **Weekly Planning: At the start of each week, review the meal plan.** Make a grocery list of the ingredients needed.
2. **Batch Cooking:** Prepare larger portions of meals that can be stored and used for multiple days, especially for lunches and dinners.
3. **Meal Prepping:** Prepare ingredients in advance, such as chopping vegetables or cooking grains, to save time during the week.

Staying Flexible

1. **Adapting to Changes:** Life can be unpredictable. If you need to eat out or miss a planned meal, don't stress. Return to the plan for the next meal.
2. **Listen to Your Body:** Pay attention to how your body responds to different foods. Adjust the plan to include more of what makes you feel good and less of what doesn't.

Nutritional Balance

1. **Hydration:** Drink plenty of water throughout the day. The smoothies and drinks included in the plan also contribute to your hydration.
2. **Healthy Fats: Incorporate avocados, nuts, seeds, and olive oil as sources of healthy fats.**
3. **Lean Proteins:** Include a variety of protein sources like chicken, turkey, fish, legumes, and tofu.

Incorporating physical activity

1. **Daily exercise:** Combine this meal plan with regular physical activity. Aim for at least 30 minutes of moderate exercise most days of the week.
2. **Active Lifestyle:** Engage in activities you enjoy, such as walking, swimming, or yoga, to enhance overall health.

Monitoring Progress

1. **Tracking: Keep a food diary to record your meals, how you feel, and any changes to your health.**
2. **Consultation: If possible, consult a healthcare provider or nutritionist regularly to monitor your progress and make adjustments as needed.**

Enjoying the journey

1. **Variety:** Embrace the variety of foods and flavors. This plan is designed not only for health but also for enjoyment.
2. **Mindful Eating:** Eat slowly and mindfully, savoring each bite. This helps with digestion and enhances the eating experience.

By following these guidelines, you can effectively use the 60-day meal plan to support your liver health, boost your vitality, and enjoy delicious, nourishing meals. Remember, this plan is a tool to help you on your health journey, so adapt it to fit your lifestyle and needs. Enjoy the process of nourishing your body with wholesome foods!

Benefits of a Structured Meal Plan

Adopting a structured meal plan offers numerous advantages, particularly when aiming to manage and improve conditions such as fatty liver disease. Here's a look at the key benefits:

1. Nutritional balance

Ensures Adequate Nutrient Intake: A structured meal plan helps ensure that you consume a well-balanced diet rich in essential nutrients. This balance is crucial for maintaining overall health and supporting liver function.

Prevents Nutrient Deficiencies: By following a meal plan, you can avoid common nutrient deficiencies. The plan incorporates a variety of foods to provide vitamins, minerals, proteins, healthy fats, and carbohydrates.

2. Supports liver health

Reduces Liver Fat: A structured meal plan designed for fatty liver disease focuses on reducing liver fat by including foods that are low in saturated fats and high in fiber, antioxidants, and healthy fats.

Promotes Liver Detoxification: Certain foods included in the plan, such as leafy greens, citrus fruits, and nuts, support the liver's natural detoxification processes.

3. Aids in Weight Management

Helps with Weight Loss: Following a structured meal plan can assist in weight loss by providing portion-controlled, calorie-conscious meals that prevent overeating and promote a healthy weight.

Maintains Healthy Weight: For those not needing to lose weight, a meal plan helps maintain a healthy weight by ensuring balanced calorie intake.

4. Simplifies meal preparation

Saves Time: A structured meal plan simplifies meal preparation by providing a clear guide on what to eat and when. This reduces time spent deciding on meals and grocery shopping.

Encourages Batch Cooking: Planning meals ahead allows for batch cooking, which can save time and reduce daily cooking stress.

5. Improves dietary habits.

Unhealthy Choices Are Reduced: With a plan in place, you are less likely to make impulsive and unhealthy food choices. This aids in consistently adhering to a healthy diet.

Promotes Consistent Eating Patterns: Structured eating schedules promote regular meal times, which can improve metabolism and overall digestive health.

6. Increases food diversity and enjoyment

Introduces New Recipes: A meal plan encourages trying new recipes and ingredients, adding variety to your diet, and preventing meal boredom.

Improves Food Relationships: Having a positive and structured approach to meals can enhance your relationship with food, making eating a more enjoyable and mindful experience.

7. Promotes overall health.

Boosts Energy Levels: Consuming balanced and nutritious meals can significantly boost your energy levels and improve overall vitality.

Enhances Mental Well-being: Good nutrition is closely linked to mental health. A well-structured meal plan can help reduce the stress and anxiety associated with meal planning, as well as improve mood and cognitive function.

8. Allows for medical and nutritional monitoring.

Easier Tracking for Health Professionals: Following a structured plan enables healthcare providers to track and monitor more easily. They can make more informed recommendations and adjustments based on a consistent dietary pattern.

Helps Identify Food Sensitivities: A structured approach can help identify any food sensitivities or allergies by systematically eliminating and reintroducing foods.

9. Cost-Effective

Reduces Food Waste: By planning meals and grocery shopping accordingly, you reduce food waste and save money on unused or spoiled food.

Encourages Budget-Friendly Choices: A meal plan helps in purchasing only what is needed, often leading to more economical choices and avoiding unnecessary expenses.

Weekly Meal Plans

Day 1:
- **Breakfast:** Spinach and Mushroom Omelet
- **Lunch:** Quinoa Salad with Chickpeas and Veggies
- **Dinner:** Baked Lemon Herb Chicken
- **Snack:** Apple Slices with Almond Butter
- **Smoothie:** Green Detox Smoothie

Day 2:
- **Breakfast:** Overnight Chia Pudding with Berries
- **Lunch:** Lentil Soup with Vegetables
- **Dinner:** Roasted Salmon with Asparagus and Potatoes
- **Snack:** Greek Yogurt with Mixed Berries
- **Smoothie:** Berry Blast Smoothie

Day 3:
- **Breakfast:** Avocado Toast with Whole Grain Bread
- **Lunch:** Grilled Vegetable Wrap
- **Dinner:** Turkey and Vegetable Stir-Fry
- **Snack:** Carrot Sticks with Hummus
- **Smoothie:** Tropical Turmeric Smoothie

Day 4:
- **Breakfast:** Greek Yogurt Parfait with Granola and Berries
- **Lunch:** Stuffed Bell Peppers with Quinoa and Black Beans
- **Dinner:** Quinoa and Black Bean Stuffed Zucchini Boats
- **Snack:** Rice Cake with Avocado
- **Smoothie:** Avocado Banana Smoothie

Day 5:

- **Breakfast:** Berry Smoothie Bowl with Nuts and Seeds
- **Lunch:** Spinach and Feta Stuffed Chicken Breast
- **Dinner:** Lentil and Vegetable Curry
- **Snack:** Cottage Cheese with Pineapple
- **Smoothie:** Beetroot Berry Smoothie

Day 6:

- **Breakfast:** Oatmeal with Fresh Fruit and Nuts
- **Lunch:** Turkey and Veggie Lettuce Wraps
- **Dinner:** Grilled Turkey Burgers with Sweet Potato Fries
- **Snack:** Trail Mix with Nuts and Dried Fruit
- **Smoothie:** Cucumber Mint Cooler

Day 7:

- **Breakfast:** Smoothie with Spinach, Banana, and Almond Milk
- **Lunch:** Roasted Vegetable and Hummus Wrap
- **Dinner:** Shrimp and Vegetable Skewers
- **Snack:** Veggie Sticks with Guacamole
- **Smoothie:** Golden Milk Latte

Day 8:

- **Breakfast:** Smoothie with Mixed Berries and Greek Yogurt
- **Lunch:** Chickpea and Avocado Salad
- **Dinner:** Vegetable and Tofu Stir-Fry
- **Snack:** Edamame Beans
- **Smoothie:** Citrus Green Tea

Day 9:

- Breakfast: Greek Yogurt with Honey and Nuts
- Lunch: Lentil Salad with Feta and Vegetables
- Dinner: Eggplant Parmesan
- Snack: Cottage Cheese and Tomato Salad
- Smoothie: Watermelon Mint Refresher

Day 10:

- Breakfast: Whole Grain Toast with Nut Butter and Banana
- Lunch: Mediterranean Chickpea Salad
- Dinner: Baked Lemon Herb Chicken
- Snack: Apple Slices with Almond Butter
- Smoothie: Peach Ginger Iced Tea

Day 11:

- Breakfast: Overnight Chia Pudding with Berries
- Lunch: Quinoa Salad with Chickpeas and Veggies
- Dinner: Roasted Salmon with Asparagus and Potatoes
- Snack: Greek Yogurt with Mixed Berries
- Smoothie: Green Detox Smoothie

Day 12:

- Breakfast: Spinach and Mushroom Omelet
- Lunch: Lentil Soup with Vegetables
- Dinner: Turkey and Vegetable Stir-Fry
- Snack: Carrot Sticks with Hummus
- Smoothie: Berry Blast Smoothie

Day 13:
- **Breakfast:** Avocado Toast with Whole Grain Bread
- Lunch: Grilled Vegetable Wrap
- Dinner: Quinoa and Black Bean Stuffed Zucchini Boats
- Snack: Rice Cake with Avocado
- Smoothie: Tropical Turmeric Smoothie

Day 14:
- Breakfast: Greek Yogurt Parfait with Granola and Berries
- Lunch: Stuffed Bell Peppers with Quinoa and Black Beans
- Dinner: Lentil and Vegetable Curry
- Snack: Cottage Cheese with Pineapple
- Smoothie: Avocado Banana Smoothie

Day 15:
- Breakfast: Berry Smoothie Bowl with Nuts and Seeds
- Lunch: Spinach and Feta Stuffed Chicken Breast
- Dinner: Grilled Turkey Burgers with Sweet Potato Fries
- Snack: Trail Mix with Nuts and Dried Fruit
- Smoothie: Beetroot Berry Smoothie

Day 16:
- Breakfast: Oatmeal with Fresh Fruit and Nuts
- Lunch: Turkey and Veggie Lettuce Wraps
- Dinner: Shrimp and Vegetable Skewers
- Snack: Veggie Sticks with Guacamole
- Smoothie: Cucumber Mint Cooler

Day 17:
- Breakfast: Greek Yogurt with Mixed Berries
- Lunch: Grilled Vegetable Wrap
- Dinner: Roasted Salmon with Asparagus and Potatoes
- Snack: Cottage Cheese and Tomato Salad
- Smoothie: Green Detox Smoothie

Day 18:
- Breakfast: Overnight Chia Pudding with Berries
- Lunch: Quinoa Salad with Chickpeas and Veggies
- Dinner: Turkey and Vegetable Stir-Fry
- Snack: Edamame Beans
- Smoothie: Berry Blast Smoothie

Day 19:
- Breakfast: Spinach and Mushroom Omelet
- Lunch: Lentil Soup with Vegetables
- Dinner: Eggplant Parmesan
- Snack: Veggie Sticks with Guacamole
- Smoothie: Tropical Turmeric Smoothie

Day 20:
- Breakfast: Avocado Toast with Whole Grain Bread
- Lunch: Roasted Vegetable and Hummus Wrap
- Dinner: Baked Lemon Herb Chicken
- Snack: Apple Slices with Almond Butter
- Smoothie: Avocado Banana Smoothie

Day 21:
- Breakfast: Greek Yogurt Parfait with Granola and Berries
- Lunch: Chickpea and Avocado Salad
- Dinner: Quinoa and Black Bean Stuffed Zucchini Boats
- Snack: Carrot Sticks with Hummus
- Smoothie: Beetroot Berry Smoothie

Day 22:
- Breakfast: Berry Smoothie Bowl with Nuts and Seeds
- Lunch: Mediterranean Chickpea Salad
- Dinner: Lentil and Vegetable Curry
- Snack: Cottage Cheese with Pineapple
- Smoothie: Cucumber Mint Cooler

Day 23:
- Breakfast: Oatmeal with Fresh Fruit and Nuts
- Lunch: Turkey and Veggie Lettuce Wraps
- Dinner: Shrimp and Vegetable Skewers
- Snack: Rice Cake with Avocado
- Smoothie: Golden Milk Latte

Day 24:
- Breakfast: Smoothie with Spinach, Banana, and Almond Milk
- Lunch: Lentil Salad with Feta and Vegetables
- Dinner: Vegetable and Tofu Stir-Fry
- Snack: Trail Mix with Nuts and Dried Fruit
- Smoothie: Citrus Green Tea

Day 25:
- Breakfast: Greek Yogurt with Honey and Nuts
- Lunch: Quinoa Salad with Chickpeas and Veggies
- Dinner: Baked Lemon Herb Chicken
- Snack: Greek Yogurt with Mixed Berries
- Smoothie: Green Detox Smoothie

Day 26:
- Breakfast: Whole Grain Toast with Nut Butter and Banana
- Lunch: Lentil Soup with Vegetables
- Dinner: Turkey and Vegetable Stir-Fry
- Snack: Carrot Sticks with Hummus
- Smoothie: Berry Blast Smoothie

Day 27:
- Breakfast: Overnight Chia Pudding with Berries
- Lunch: Grilled Vegetable Wrap
- Dinner: Eggplant Parmesan
- Snack: Cottage Cheese and Tomato Salad
- Smoothie: Tropical Turmeric Smoothie

Day 28:
- Breakfast: Spinach and Mushroom Omelet
- Lunch: Roasted Vegetable and Hummus Wrap
- Dinner: Baked Lemon Herb Chicken
- Snack: Apple Slices with Almond Butter
- Smoothie: Avocado Banana Smoothie

Day 29:
- Breakfast: Avocado Toast with Whole Grain Bread
- Lunch: Chickpea and Avocado Salad
- Dinner: Quinoa and Black Bean Stuffed Zucchini Boats
- Snack: Edamame Beans
- Smoothie: Beetroot Berry Smoothie

Day 30:
- Breakfast: Greek Yogurt Parfait with Granola and Berries
- Lunch: Mediterranean Chickpea Salad
- Dinner: Lentil and Vegetable Curry
- Snack: Veggie Sticks with Guacamole
- Smoothie: Cucumber Mint Cooler

Day 31:
- Breakfast: Berry Smoothie Bowl with Nuts and Seeds
- Lunch: Spinach and Feta Stuffed Chicken Breast
- Dinner: Shrimp and Vegetable Skewers
- Snack: Cottage Cheese with Pineapple
- Smoothie: Golden Milk Latte

Day 32:
- Breakfast: Oatmeal with Fresh Fruit and Nuts
- Lunch: Turkey and Veggie Lettuce Wraps
- Dinner: Vegetable and Tofu Stir-Fry
- Snack: Trail Mix with Nuts and Dried Fruit
- Smoothie: Citrus Green Tea

Day 33:
- Breakfast: Smoothie with Spinach, Banana, and Almond Milk
- Lunch: Lentil Salad with Feta and Vegetables
- Dinner: Baked Lemon Herb Chicken
- Snack: Greek Yogurt with Mixed Berries
- Smoothie: Green Detox Smoothie

Day 34:
- Breakfast: Greek Yogurt with Honey and Nuts
- Lunch: Quinoa Salad with Chickpeas and Veggies
- Dinner: Turkey and Vegetable Stir-Fry
- Snack: Carrot Sticks with Hummus
- Smoothie: Berry Blast Smoothie

Day 35:
- Breakfast: Whole Grain Toast with Nut Butter and Banana
- Lunch: Lentil Soup with Vegetables
- Dinner: Eggplant Parmesan
- Snack: Cottage Cheese and Tomato Salad
- Smoothie: Tropical Turmeric Smoothie

Day 36:
- Breakfast: Overnight Chia Pudding with Berries
- Lunch: Grilled Vegetable Wrap
- Dinner: Baked Lemon Herb Chicken
- Snack: Apple Slices with Almond Butter
- Smoothie: Avocado Banana Smoothie

Day 37:
- **Breakfast:** Spinach and Mushroom Omelet
- **Lunch:** Roasted Vegetable and Hummus Wrap
- **Dinner:** Quinoa and Black Bean Stuffed Zucchini Boats
- **Snack:** Edamame Beans
- **Smoothie:** Beetroot Berry Smoothie

Day 38:
- **Breakfast:** Avocado Toast with Whole Grain Bread
- **Lunch:** Chickpea and Avocado Salad
- **Dinner:** Lentil and Vegetable Curry
- **Snack:** Veggie Sticks with Guacamole
- **Smoothie:** Cucumber Mint Cooler

Day 39:
- Breakfast: Greek Yogurt Parfait with Granola and Berries
- Lunch: Mediterranean Chickpea Salad
- Dinner: Shrimp and Vegetable Skewers
- Snack: Cottage Cheese with Pineapple
- Smoothie: Golden Milk Latte

Day 40:
- **Breakfast:** Berry Smoothie Bowl with Nuts and Seeds
- **Lunch:** Spinach and Feta Stuffed Chicken Breast
- **Dinner:** Vegetable and Tofu Stir-Fry
- **Snack:** Trail Mix with Nuts and Dried Fruit
- **Smoothie:** Citrus Green Tea

Day 41:
- **Breakfast:** Oatmeal with Fresh Fruit and Nuts
- **Lunch:** Turkey and Veggie Lettuce Wraps
- **Dinner:** Baked Lemon Herb Chicken
- **Snack:** Greek Yogurt with Mixed Berries
- **Smoothie:** Green Detox Smoothie

Day 42:
- Breakfast: Smoothie with Spinach, Banana, and Almond Milk
- Lunch: Lentil Salad with Feta and Vegetables
- Dinner: Turkey and Vegetable Stir-Fry
- Snack: Carrot Sticks with Hummus
- Smoothie: Berry Blast Smoothie

Day 43:

- Breakfast: Greek Yogurt with Honey and Nuts
- Lunch: Quinoa Salad with Chickpeas and Veggies
- Dinner: Eggplant Parmesan
- Snack: Cottage Cheese and Tomato Salad
- Smoothie: Tropical Turmeric Smoothie

Day 44:

- Breakfast: Whole Grain Toast with Nut Butter and Banana
- Lunch: Lentil Soup with Vegetables
- Dinner: Baked Lemon Herb Chicken
- Snack: Apple Slices with Almond Butter
- Smoothie: Avocado Banana Smoothie

Day 45:

- Breakfast: Overnight Chia Pudding with Berries
- Lunch: Grilled Vegetable Wrap
- Dinner: Quinoa and Black Bean Stuffed Zucchini Boats
- Snack: Edamame Beans
- Smoothie: Beetroot Berry Smoothie

Day 46:

- Breakfast: Spinach and Mushroom Omelet
- Lunch: Roasted Vegetable and Hummus Wrap
- Dinner: Lentil and Vegetable Curry
- Snack: Veggie Sticks with Guacamole
- Smoothie: Cucumber Mint Cooler

Day 47:

- Breakfast: Avocado Toast with Whole Grain Bread
- Lunch: Chickpea and Avocado Salad
- Dinner: Shrimp and Vegetable Skewers
- Snack: Cottage Cheese with Pineapple
- Smoothie: Golden Milk Latte

Day 48:

- Breakfast: Greek Yogurt Parfait with Granola and Berries
- Lunch: Mediterranean Chickpea Salad
- Dinner: Vegetable and Tofu Stir-Fry
- Snack: Trail Mix with Nuts and Dried Fruit
- Smoothie: Citrus Green Tea

Day 49:

- Breakfast: Avocado Toast with Whole Grain Bread
- Lunch: Grilled Vegetable Wrap
- Dinner: Quinoa and Black Bean Stuffed Zucchini Boats
- Snack: Rice Cake with Avocado
- Smoothie: Tropical Turmeric Smoothie

Day 50:

- Breakfast: Greek Yogurt Parfait with Granola and Berries
- Lunch: Stuffed Bell Peppers with Quinoa and Black Beans
- Dinner: Lentil and Vegetable Curry
- Snack: Cottage Cheese with Pineapple
- Smoothie: Avocado Banana Smoothie

Day 51:

- Breakfast: Berry Smoothie Bowl with Nuts and Seeds
- Lunch: Spinach and Feta Stuffed Chicken Breast
- Dinner: Grilled Turkey Burgers with Sweet Potato Fries
- Snack: Trail Mix with Nuts and Dried Fruit
- Smoothie: Beetroot Berry Smoothie

Day 53:

- Breakfast: Oatmeal with Fresh Fruit and Nuts
- Lunch: Turkey and Veggie Lettuce Wraps
- Dinner: Shrimp and Vegetable Skewers
- Snack: Veggie Sticks with Guacamole
- Smoothie: Cucumber Mint Cooler

Day 54:

- Breakfast: Greek Yogurt with Mixed Berries
- Lunch: Grilled Vegetable Wrap
- Dinner: Roasted Salmon with Asparagus and Potatoes
- Snack: Cottage Cheese and Tomato Salad
- Smoothie: Green Detox Smoothie

Day 55:

- Breakfast: Overnight Chia Pudding with Berries
- Lunch: Quinoa Salad with Chickpeas and Veggies
- Dinner: Turkey and Vegetable Stir-Fry
- Snack: Edamame Beans
- Smoothie: Berry Blast Smoothie

Day 56:
- **Breakfast:** Spinach and Mushroom Omelet
- **Lunch:** Lentil Soup with Vegetables
- **Dinner:** Eggplant Parmesan
- **Snack:** Veggie Sticks with Guacamole
- **Smoothie:** Tropical Turmeric Smoothie

Day 59:
- **Breakfast:** Avocado Toast with Whole Grain Bread
- **Lunch:** Roasted Vegetable and Hummus Wrap
- **Dinner:** Baked Lemon Herb Chicken

- **Snack:** Apple Slices with Almond Butter
- **Smoothie:** Avocado Banana Smoothie

Day 60:
- **Breakfast:** Greek Yogurt Parfait with Granola and Berries
- **Lunch:** Chickpea and Avocado Salad
- **Dinner:** Quinoa and Black Bean Stuffed Zucchini Boats
- **Snack:** Carrot Sticks with Hummus
- **Smoothie:** Beetroot Berry Smoothie

Shopping Lists

Weekly Shopping Lists for Easy Planning

Week 1 Shopping List

Produce:

- **Spinach (2 bunches)**
- **Avocados (5)**
- **Bananas (7)**
- **Blueberries (2 cups)**
- **Strawberries (2 cups)**
- **Mixed Greens (1 large bag)**
- **Tomatoes (6)**
- **Broccoli (2 heads)**
- **Asparagus (1 bunch)**
- **Sweet Potatoes (4)**
- **Zucchini (4)**
- **Bell Peppers (6)**
- **Carrots (1 bag)**
- **Cucumbers (4)**
- **Apples (7)**
- **Mixed Berries (1 bag)**
- **Mint (1 bunch)**
- **Kale (1 bunch)**
- **Pineapple (1)**
- **Pomegranate (1)**
- **Beetroot (2)**

Protein:

- **Greek Yogurt (1 large tub)**
- **Eggs (2 dozen)**
- **Chicken Breast (4 fillets)**
- **Salmon (4 fillets)**
- **Cod (4 fillets)**
- **Turkey (ground, 1 lb)**
- **Tofu (2 blocks)**
- **Shrimp (1 lb)**
- **Black Beans (1 can)**
- **Chickpeas (1 can)**
- **Tuna (2 cans)**
- **Edamame (1 bag, frozen)**
- **Walnuts (1 bag)**
- **Mixed Nuts (1 bag)**

Grains & Seeds:

- **Whole Grain Bread (1 loaf)**
- **Quinoa (1 lb)**
- **Brown Rice (1 lb)**
- **Chia Seeds (1 bag)**
- **Oats (1 lb)**
- **Flaxseeds (1 bag)**
- **Rice Cakes (1 pack)**

Dairy & Alternatives:

- **Almond Milk (1 quart)**
- **Coconut Milk (1 can)**
- **Feta Cheese (1 block)**
- **Hummus (1 tub)**
- **Cheese (your choice, 1 block)**

Pantry Staples:

- **Olive Oil (1 bottle)**
- **Almond Butter (1 jar)**
- **Honey (1 jar)**
- **Lemon Juice (1 bottle)**
- **Balsamic Vinegar (1 bottle)**
- **Soy Sauce (1 bottle)**
- **Paprika (1 jar)**
- **Sea Salt (1 jar)**

Frozen:

- Mixed Vegetables (1 bag)

Week 2 Shopping List

Produce:

- **Spinach (2 bunches)**
- **Avocados (5)**
- **Blueberries (2 cups)**
- **Mixed Greens (1 large bag)**
- **Tomatoes (6)**
- **Carrots (1 bag)**
- **Cucumbers (4)**
- **Apples (7)**
- **Pineapple (1)**
- **Mixed Berries (1 bag)**
- **Mint (1 bunch)**
- **Kale (1 bunch)**
- **Bananas (7)**
- **Strawberries (2 cups)**
- **Broccoli (2 heads)**
- **Asparagus (1 bunch)**
- **Sweet Potatoes (4)**
- **Zucchini (4)**
- **Bell Peppers (6)**
- **Mango (2)**
- **Lemons (4)**
- **Oranges (6)**
- **Ginger (1 small root)**

Protein:

- **Greek Yogurt (1 large tub)**
- **Eggs (2 dozen)**
- **Chicken Breast (4 fillets)**
- **Salmon (4 fillets)**
- **Cod (4 fillets)**
- **Turkey (ground, 1 lb)**
- **Tofu (2 blocks)**
- **Shrimp (1 lb)**

- **Black Beans (1 can)**
- **Chickpeas (1 can)**
- **Tuna (2 cans)**
- **Walnuts (1 bag)**
- **Mixed Nuts (1 bag)**
- **Almond Butter (1 jar)**
- **Chia Seeds (1 bag)**
- **Oats (1 lb)**
- **Flaxseeds (1 bag)**
- **Rice Cakes (1 pack)**
- **Lentils (1 lb)**
- **Edamame (1 bag, frozen)**

Grains & Seeds:

- **Whole Grain Bread (1 loaf)**
- **Quinoa (1 lb)**
- **Brown Rice (1 lb)**

Dairy & Alternatives:

- **Almond Milk (1 quart)**
- **Coconut Milk (1 can)**
- **Feta Cheese (1 block)**
- **Hummus (1 tub)**

Pantry Staples:

- **Olive Oil (1 bottle)**
- **Honey (1 jar)**
- **Lemon Juice (1 bottle)**
- **Balsamic Vinegar (1 bottle)**
- **Soy Sauce (1 bottle)**
- **Paprika (1 jar)**
- **Sea Salt (1 jar)**

Frozen:

- **Mixed Vegetables (1 bag)**

Week 3 Shopping List

Produce:

- **Spinach (2 bunches)**
- **Avocados (5)**

- Blueberries (2 cups)
- Mixed Greens (1 large bag)
- Tomatoes (6)
- Carrots (1 bag)
- Cucumbers (4)
- Apples (7)
- Pineapple (1)
- Mixed Berries (1 bag)
- Mint (1 bunch)
- Kale (1 bunch)
- Bananas (7)
- Strawberries (2 cups)
- Broccoli (2 heads)
- Asparagus (1 bunch)
- Sweet Potatoes (4)
- Zucchini (4)
- Bell Peppers (6)
- Mango (2)
- Lemons (4)
- Oranges (6)
- Ginger (1 small root)
- Pomegranate (1)
- Beetroot (2)

Protein:

- Greek Yogurt (1 large tub)
- Eggs (2 dozen)
- Chicken Breast (4 fillets)
- Salmon (4 fillets)
- Cod (4 fillets)
- Turkey (ground, 1 lb)
- Tofu (2 blocks)
- Shrimp (1 lb)
- Black Beans (1 can)
- Chickpeas (1 can)
- Tuna (2 cans)

- Walnuts (1 bag)
- Mixed Nuts (1 bag)
- Almond Butter (1 jar)
- Chia Seeds (1 bag)
- Oats (1 lb)
- Flaxseeds (1 bag)
- Rice Cakes (1 pack)
- Lentils (1 lb)
- Edamame (1 bag, frozen)

Grains & Seeds:

- Whole Grain Bread (1 loaf)
- Quinoa (1 lb)
- Brown Rice (1 lb)

Dairy & Alternatives:

- Almond Milk (1 quart)
- Coconut Milk (1 can)
- Feta Cheese (1 block)
- Hummus (1 tub)

Pantry Staples:

- Olive Oil (1 bottle)
- Honey (1 jar)
- Lemon Juice (1 bottle)
- Balsamic Vinegar (1 bottle)
- Soy Sauce (1 bottle)
- Paprika (1 jar)
- Sea Salt (1 jar)

Frozen:

- Mixed Vegetables (1 bag)

Week 4 Shopping List

Produce:

- Spinach (2 bunches)
- Avocados (5)
- Blueberries (2 cups)
- Mixed Greens (1 large bag)
- Tomatoes (6)

- Carrots (1 bag)
- Cucumbers (4)
- Apples (7)
- Pineapple (1)
- Mixed Berries (1 bag)
- Mint (1 bunch)
- Kale (1 bunch)
- Bananas (7)
- Strawberries (2 cups)
- Broccoli (2 heads)
- Asparagus (1 bunch)
- Sweet Potatoes (4)
- Zucchini (4)
- Bell Peppers (6)
- Mango (2)
- Lemons (4)
- Oranges (6)
- Ginger (1 small root)
- Pomegranate (1)
- Beetroot (2)

Protein:

- Greek Yogurt (1 large tub)
- Eggs (2 dozen)
- Chicken Breast (4 fillets)
- Salmon (4 fillets)
- Cod (4 fillets)
- Turkey (ground, 1 lb)
- Tofu (2 blocks)
- Shrimp (1 lb)
- Black Beans (1 can)
- Chickpeas (1 can)
- Tuna (2 cans)
- Walnuts (1 bag)
- Mixed Nuts (1 bag)
- Almond Butter (1 jar)
- Chia Seeds (1 bag)
- Oats (1 lb)
- Flaxseeds (1 bag)
- Rice Cakes (1 pack)
- Lentils (1 lb)
- Edamame (1 bag, frozen)

Grains & Seeds:

- Whole Grain Bread (1 loaf)
- Quinoa (1 lb)
- Brown Rice (1 lb)

Dairy & Alternatives:

- Almond Milk (1 quart)
- Coconut Milk (1 can)
- Feta Cheese (1 block)
- Hummus (1 tub)

Pantry Staples:

- Olive Oil (1 bottle)
- Honey (1 jar)
- Lemon Juice (1 bottle)
- Balsamic Vinegar (1 bottle)
- Soy Sauce (1 bottle)
- Paprika (1 jar)
- Sea Salt (1 jar)

Frozen:

- Mixed Vegetables (1 bag)

Week 5 Shopping List

Produce:

- Spinach (2 bunches)
- Avocados (5)
- Blueberries (2 cups)
- Mixed Greens (1 large bag)
- Tomatoes (6)
- Carrots (1 bag)
- Cucumbers (4)
- Apples (7)

- **Pineapple (1)**
- **Mixed Berries (1 bag)**
- **Mint (1 bunch)**
- **Kale (1 bunch)**
- **Bananas (7)**
- **Strawberries (2 cups)**
- **Broccoli (2 heads)**
- **Asparagus (1 bunch)**
- **Sweet Potatoes (4)**
- **Zucchini (4)**
- **Bell Peppers (6)**
- **Mango (2)**
- **Lemons (4)**
- **Oranges (6)**
- **Ginger (1 small root)**
- **Pomegranate (1)**
- **Beetroot (2)**

Protein:
- **Greek Yogurt (1 large tub)**
- **Eggs (2 dozen)**
- **Chicken Breast (4 fillets)**
- **Salmon (4 fillets)**
- **Cod (4 fillets)**
- **Turkey (ground, 1 lb)**
- **Tofu (2 blocks)**
- **Shrimp (1 lb)**
- **Black Beans (1 can)**
- **Chickpeas (1 can)**
- **Tuna (2 cans)**
- **Walnuts (1 bag)**
- **Mixed Nuts (1 bag)**
- **Almond Butter (1 jar)**
- **Chia Seeds (1 bag)**
- **Oats (1 lb)**
- **Flaxseeds (1 bag)**

- **Rice Cakes (1 pack)**
- **Lentils (1 lb)**
- **Edamame (1 bag, frozen)**

Grains & Seeds:
- **Whole Grain Bread (1 loaf)**
- **Quinoa (1 lb)**
- **Brown Rice (1 lb)**

Dairy & Alternatives:
- **Almond Milk (1 quart)**
- **Coconut Milk (1 can)**
- **Feta Cheese (1 block)**
- **Hummus (1 tub)**

Pantry Staples:
- **Olive Oil (1 bottle)**
- **Honey (1 jar)**
- **Lemon Juice (1 bottle)**
- **Balsamic Vinegar (1 bottle)**
- **Soy Sauce (1 bottle)**
- **Paprika (1 jar)**
- **Sea Salt (1 jar)**

Frozen:
- **Mixed Vegetables (1 bag)**

Week 6 Shopping List

Produce:
- **Spinach (2 bunches)**
- **Avocados (5)**
- **Blueberries (2 cups)**
- **Mixed Greens (1 large bag)**
- **Tomatoes (6)**
- **Carrots (1 bag)**
- **Cucumbers (4)**
- **Apples (7)**
- **Pineapple (1)**
- **Mixed Berries (1 bag)**
- **Mint (1 bunch)**

- Kale (1 bunch)
- Bananas (7)
- Strawberries (2 cups)
- Broccoli (2 heads)
- Asparagus (1 bunch)
- Sweet Potatoes (4)
- Zucchini (4)
- Bell Peppers (6)
- Mango (2)
- Lemons (4)
- Oranges (6)
- Ginger (1 small root)
- Pomegranate (1)
- Beetroot (2)

Protein:

- Greek Yogurt (1 large tub)
- Eggs (2 dozen)
- Chicken Breast (4 fillets)
- Salmon (4 fillets)
- Cod (4 fillets)
- Turkey (ground, 1 lb)
- Tofu (2 blocks)
- Shrimp (1 lb)
- Black Beans (1 can)
- Chickpeas (1 can)
- Tuna (2 cans)
- Walnuts (1 bag)
- Mixed Nuts (1 bag)
- Almond Butter (1 jar)
- Chia Seeds (1 bag)
- Oats (1 lb)
- Flaxseeds (1 bag)
- Rice Cakes (1 pack)
- Lentils (1 lb)
- Edamame (1 bag, frozen)

Grains & Seeds:

- Whole Grain Bread (1 loaf)
- Quinoa (1 lb)
- Brown Rice (1 lb)

Dairy & Alternatives:

- Almond Milk (1 quart)
- Coconut Milk (1 can)
- Feta Cheese (1 block)
- Hummus (1 tub)

Pantry Staples:

- Olive Oil (1 bottle)
- Honey (1 jar)
- Lemon Juice (1 bottle)
- Balsamic Vinegar (1 bottle)
- Soy Sauce (1 bottle)
- Paprika (1 jar)
- Sea Salt (1 jar)

Frozen:

- Mixed Vegetables (1 bag)

Chapter 3: Breakfast Recipes

Avocado and Egg Breakfast Bowl

Prep Time: 10 minutes — Cook Time: 5 minutes — Serving Size: 1 bowl

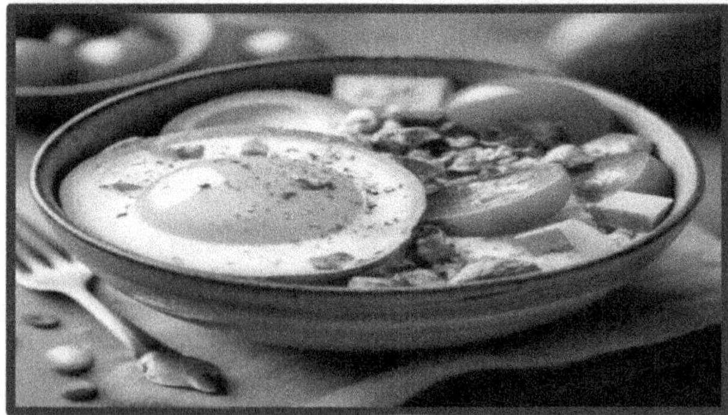

PREPARATION

Slice avocado and halve cherry tomatoes. Sauté spinach in olive oil. Cook eggs to your preference (poached, fried, or scrambled).

INGREDIENTS

Avocado, eggs, cherry tomatoes, spinach, olive oil, salt, pepper.

Nutritional Information: High in healthy fats, protein, and fiber.

Oatmeal with Berries and Almonds

Prep Time: 5 minutes — Cook Time: 5 minutes — Serving Size: 1 bowl

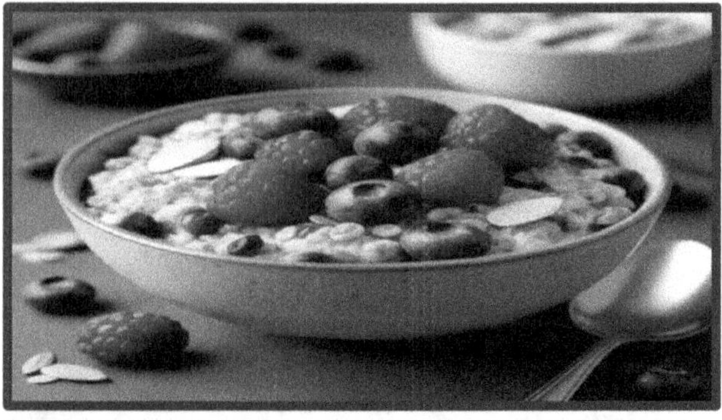

PREPARATION

Cook oats in almond milk according to package instructions. Top with mixed berries and chopped almonds. Drizzle with honey if desired.

INGREDIENTS

Rolled oats, almond milk, mixed berries, almonds, honey (optional).

Nutritional Information: High in fiber, antioxidants, and healthy fats

Greek Yogurt Parfait

Prep Time: 5 minutes | Cook Time: minutes | Serving Size: 1 parfait

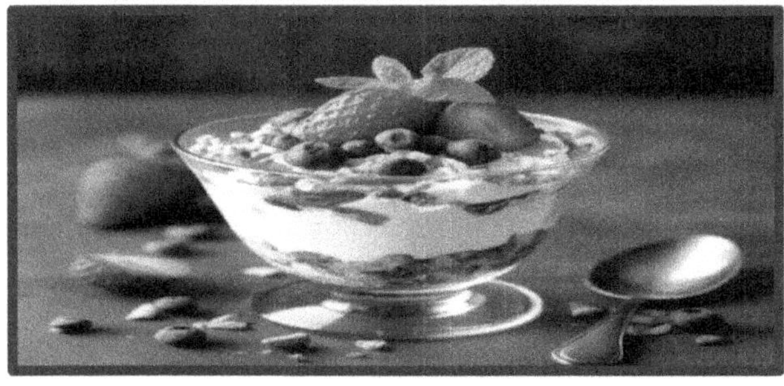

PREPARATION

Layer Greek yogurt, granola, and mixed berries in a glass or bowl. Drizzle with honey if desired.

INGREDIENTS

Greek yogurt, granola, mixed berries, honey (optional).

Nutritional Information: High in protein, probiotics, and antioxidants

Spinach and Feta Omelette

Prep Time: 5 minutes | Cook Time: 5 minutes | Serving Size: 1 omelette

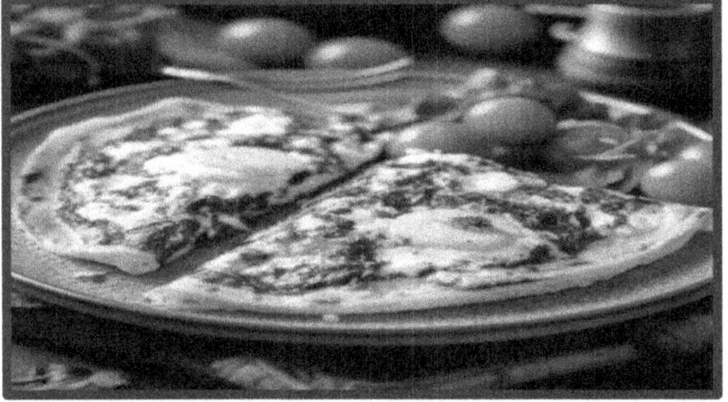

PREPARATION

Sauté spinach in olive oil until wilted. Whisk eggs and pour into a heated skillet. Add spinach and crumbled feta. Cook until set, then fold over.

INGREDIENTS

Eggs, spinach, feta cheese, olive oil, salt, pepper.

Nutritional Information: High in protein, vitamins, and minerals

Whole Grain Toast with Smashed Avocado

Prep Time: 5 minutes | Cook Time: 2 minutes | Serving Size: 2 slices

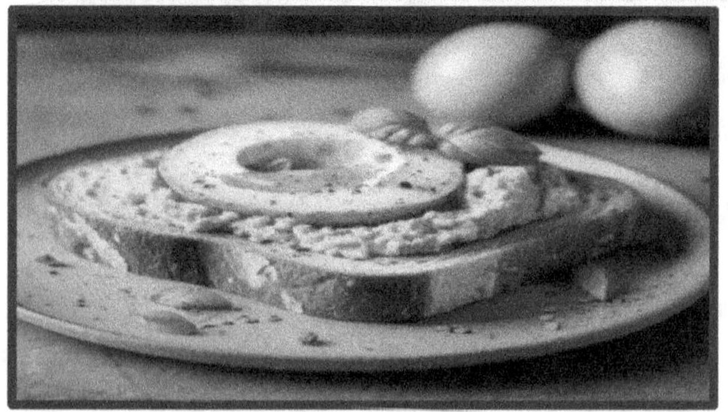

PREPARATION

Toast bread. Mash avocado with lemon juice, salt, pepper, and red pepper flakes. Spread onto toast.

INGREDIENTS

Whole grain bread, avocado, lemon juice, salt, pepper, red pepper flakes (optional).

Nutritional Information: High in fiber, healthy fats, and vitamins.

Chia Seed Pudding with Mango

Prep Time: 5 minutes (+ overnight soaking) | Cook Time: 0 minutes | Serving Size: 1 jar

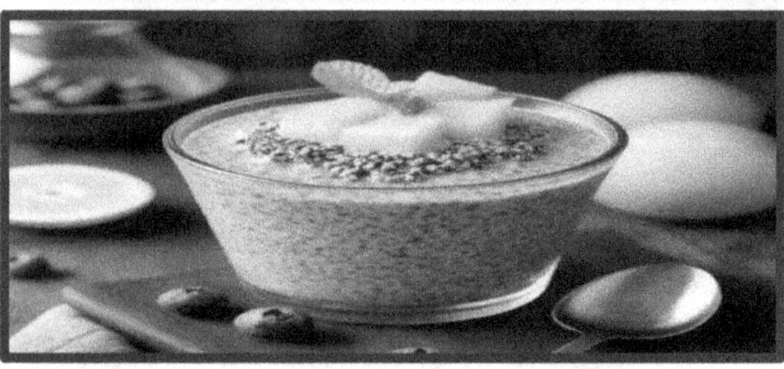

PREPARATION

Mix chia seeds and almond milk in a jar. Let sit in the fridge overnight. Top with diced mango before serving. Drizzle with honey if desired.
Nutritional Information: High in fiber, omega-3 fatty acids, and antioxidants.

INGREDIENTS

Chia seeds, almond milk, mango, honey (optional).

Nutritional Information: High in fiber, omega-3 fatty acids, and antioxidants.

Cottage Cheese and Fruit Bowl

Prep Time: 5 minutes | Cook Time: 0 minutes | Serving Size: 1 bowl

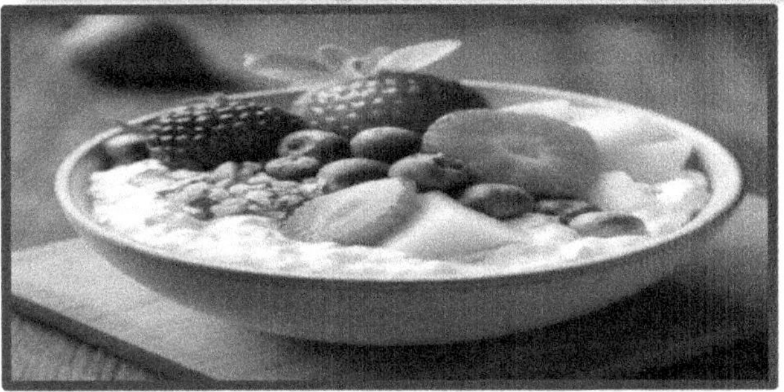

INGREDIENTS

Cottage cheese, mixed fruit (such as pineapple, kiwi, and berries), honey (optional).

PREPARATION

Dice fruit and mix with cottage cheese in a bowl. Drizzle with honey if desired.

Nutritional Information: High in protein, calcium, and vitamins.

Sweet Potato Breakfast Hash

Prep Time: 10 minutes | Cook Time: 15 minutes | Serving Size: 1 bowl

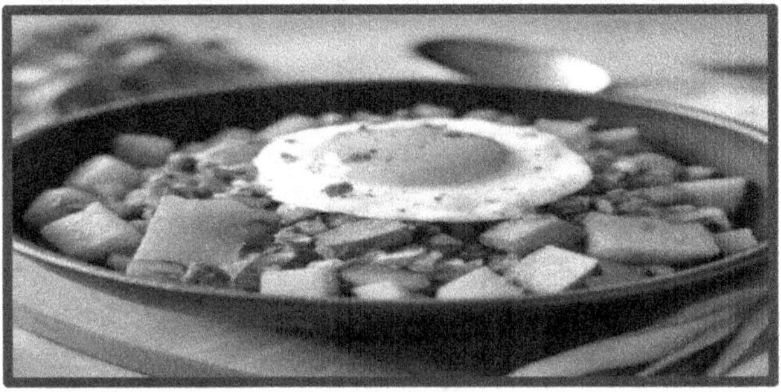

INGREDIENTS

Sweet potatoes, bell peppers, onion, turkey sausage (optional), olive oil, salt, pepper.

PREPARATION

Dice sweet potatoes, bell peppers, and onion. Sauté in olive oil until tender. Add cooked turkey sausage if desired. Season with salt and pepper.

Nutritional Information: High in fiber, vitamins, and minerals.

Quinoa Breakfast Bowl

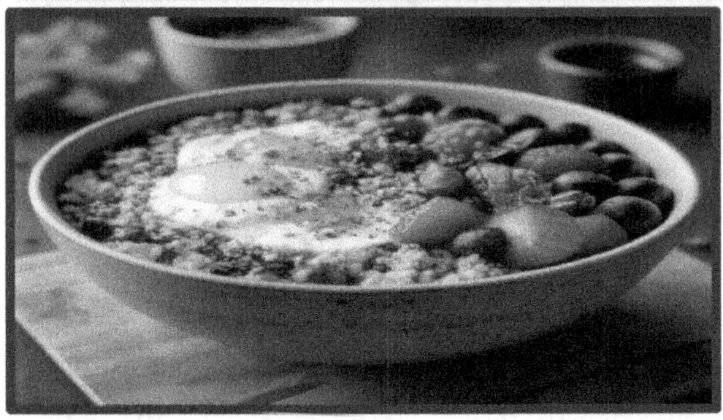

INGREDIENTS

Cooked quinoa, almond milk, cinnamon, sliced banana, chopped nuts, honey (optional).

PREPARATION

Cook quinoa in almond milk with cinnamon. Top with sliced banana, chopped nuts, and a drizzle of honey if desired.

Nutritional Information: High in protein, fiber, and essential amino acids.

Veggie Breakfast Burrito

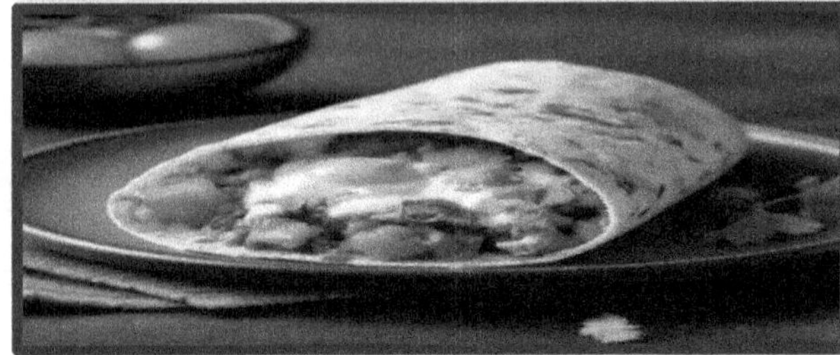

INGREDIENTS

Whole grain tortilla, scrambled eggs, black beans, diced tomatoes, spinach, avocado, salsa.

PREPARATION

Fill tortilla with scrambled eggs, black beans, diced tomatoes, spinach, and sliced avocado. Roll up and serve with salsa.

Nutritional Information: High in protein, fiber, and vitamins.

Chapter 4 Lunch Recipes

Grilled Salmon with Quinoa Salad

Prep Time: 10 minutes Cook Time: 15 minutes Serving Size: 1 fillet of salmon with quinoa salad

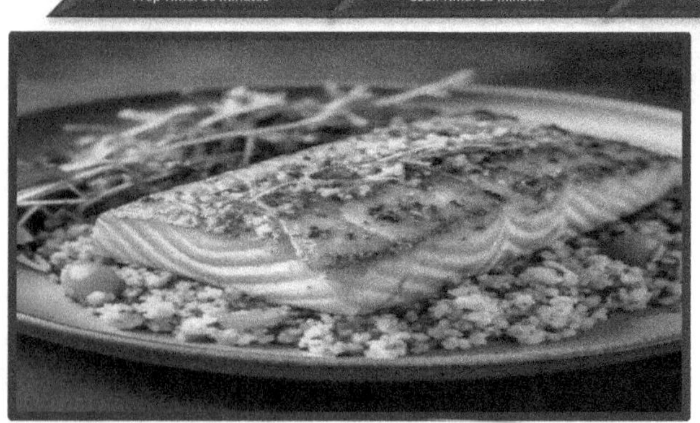

PREPARATION

Grill salmon until cooked through. Cook quinoa according to package instructions. Toss mixed greens, cucumber, and cherry tomatoes with lemon juice and olive oil. Serve grilled salmon over quinoa salad.

INGREDIENTS

Salmon fillet, quinoa, mixed greens, cucumber, cherry tomatoes, lemon, olive oil, salt, pepper.

Nutritional Information: High in omega-3 fatty acids, protein, fiber, and vitamins.

Turkey and Avocado Wrap

Prep Time: 5 minutes Cook Time: 0 minutes Serving Size: 1 wrap.

PREPARATION

Lay out wrap and layer with turkey slices, sliced avocado, lettuce, tomato, and a drizzle of mustard. Roll up tightly and slice in half.

INGREDIENTS

Whole grain wrap, roasted turkey breast slices, avocado, lettuce, tomato, mustard.

Nutritional Information: High in protein, healthy fats, fiber, and vitamins.

Quinoa and Black Bean Stuffed Bell Peppers

Prep Time: 15 minutes | Cook Time: 25 minutes | Serving Size: 1 stuffed bell pepper.

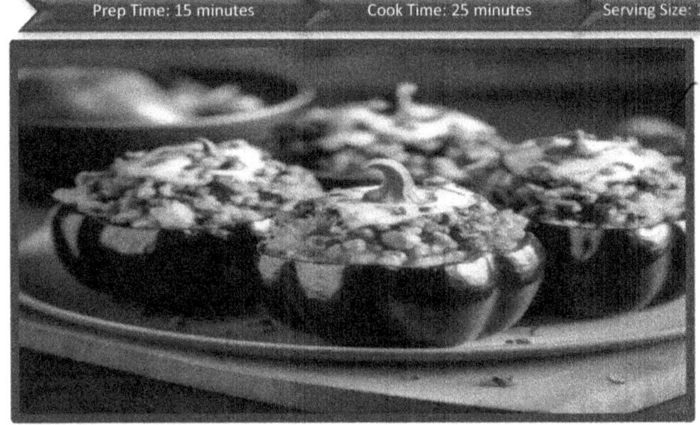

INGREDIENTS

Bell peppers, quinoa, black beans, corn, onion, garlic, cumin, chili powder, salsa, shredded cheese (optional).

PREPARATION

Cut tops off bell peppers and remove seeds. Cook quinoa according to package instructions. Sauté onion and garlic until softened, then add cooked quinoa, black beans, corn, cumin, and chili powder. Stuff mixture into bell peppers and bake until peppers are tender. Serve with salsa and shredded cheese if desired.

Nutritional Information: High in protein, fiber, vitamins, and minerals.

Chicken and Vegetable Stir-Fry

Prep Time: 15 minutes | Cook Time: 15 minutes | Serving Size: 1 serving of stir-fry with rice.

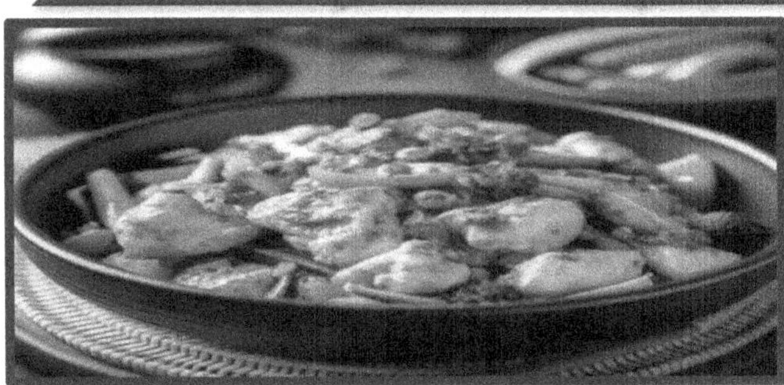

PREPARATION

Slice chicken breast into strips and marinate in soy sauce, garlic, and ginger. Stir-fry chicken and vegetables in olive oil until cooked through. Serve over cooked brown rice.

INGREDIENTS

Chicken breast, mixed vegetables (such as broccoli, bell peppers, snap peas), garlic, ginger, soy sauce, olive oil, brown rice.

Nutritional Information: High in protein, fiber, vitamins, and antioxidants.

Lentil and Vegetable Soup

Prep Time: 10 minutes   Cook Time: 30 minutes   Serving Size: 1 bowl of soup.

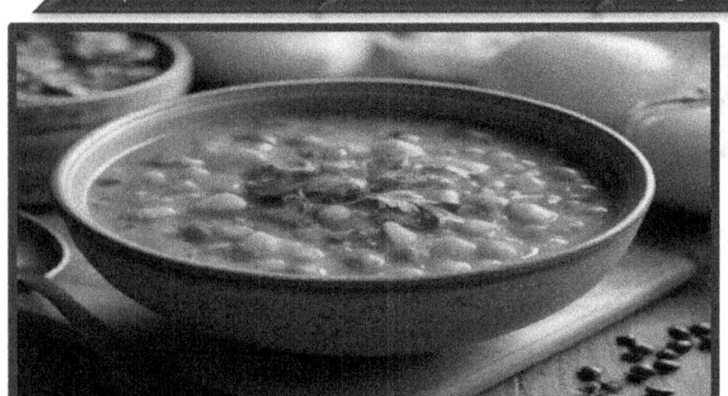

PREPARATION

Sauté onion, garlic, carrots, and celery in olive oil until softened. Add lentils, vegetable broth, thyme, and bay leaves. Simmer until lentils are tender. Stir in spinach and season with salt and pepper.

INGREDIENTS

Lentils, carrots, celery, onion, garlic, vegetable broth, spinach, thyme, bay leaves, olive oil, salt, pepper.

Nutritional Information: High in fiber, protein, vitamins, and minerals

Tuna Salad Lettuce Wraps

Prep Time: 10 minutes   Cook Time: 0 minutes   Serving Size: 1 serving of lettuce wraps.

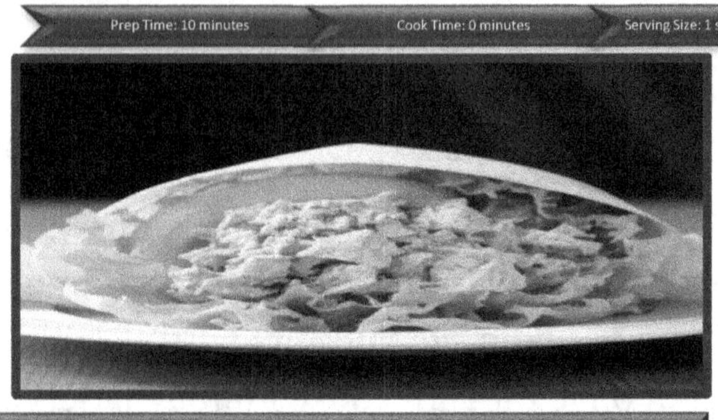

PREPARATION

Mix tuna with Greek yogurt, diced celery, red onion, lemon juice, and Dijon mustard. Spoon tuna salad onto lettuce leaves and wrap up to serve.

INGREDIENTS

Canned tuna, Greek yogurt, celery, red onion, lemon juice, Dijon mustard, lettuce leaves.

Nutritional Information: High in protein, omega-3 fatty acids, fiber, and vitamins.

Chickpea and Avocado Salad

Prep Time: 10 minutes | Cook Time: 0 minutes | Serving Size: 1 bowl of salad.

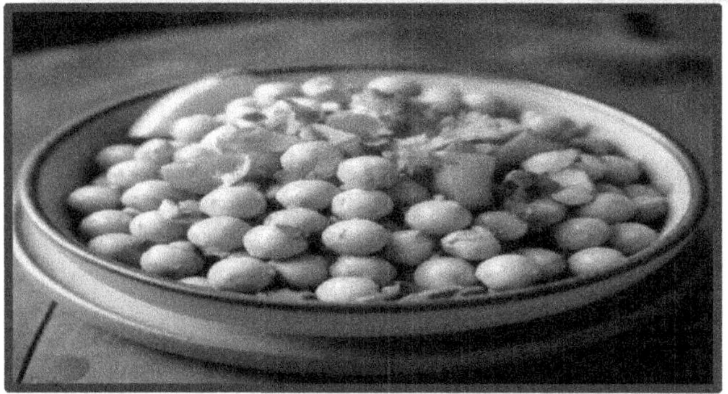

PREPARATION

Rinse and drain chickpeas. Dice avocado, cucumber, cherry tomatoes, and red onion. Toss together with chickpeas, chopped parsley, lemon juice, olive oil, salt, and pepper.

INGREDIENTS

Chickpeas, avocado, cucumber, cherry tomatoes, red onion, parsley, lemon juice, olive oil, salt, pepper.

Nutritional Information: High in fiber, protein, healthy fats, and vitamins.

Veggie and Hummus Wrap

Prep Time: 5 minutes | Cook Time: 0 minutes | Serving Size: 1 wrap.

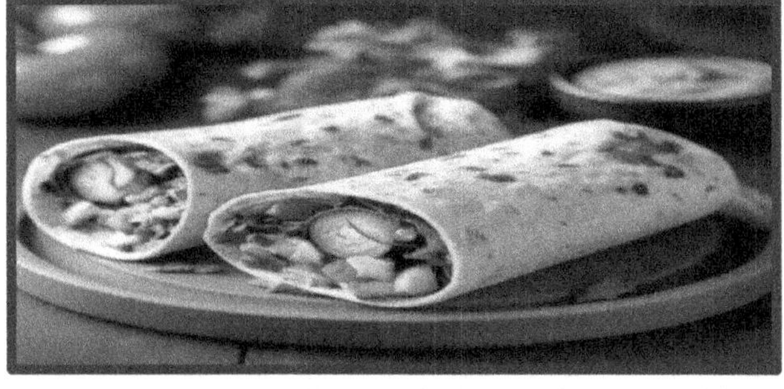

PREPARATION

Spread hummus onto wrap and layer with baby spinach, shredded carrots, sliced cucumber, and thinly sliced bell pepper. Roll up tightly and slice in half.

INGREDIENTS

Whole grain wrap, hummus, baby spinach, shredded carrots, cucumber, bell pepper.

Nutritional Information: High in fiber, protein, vitamins, and minerals.

Eggplant and Chickpea Curry

Prep Time: 15minutes | Cook Time: 25 minutes | Serving Size: 1 serving of curry.

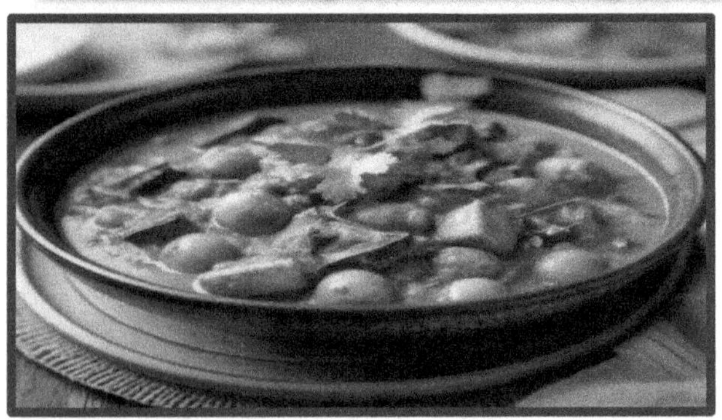

INGREDIENTS

Eggplant, chickpeas, onion, garlic, ginger, tomato sauce, coconut milk, curry powder, turmeric, cilantro, olive oil, salt, pepper.

PREPARATION

Sauté onion, garlic, and ginger in olive oil until fragrant. Add diced eggplant and cook until softened. Stir in chickpeas, tomato sauce, coconut milk, and spices. Simmer until flavors meld together. Garnish with fresh cilantro before serving.

Nutritional Information: High in fiber, protein, antioxidants, and vitamins.

Nutritional Information: High in fiber, protein, antioxidants, and vitamins.

Baked Sweet Potato with Black Bean Salsa

Prep Time: 10 minutes | Cook Time:45 minutes | Serving Size: 1 baked sweet potato with salsa.

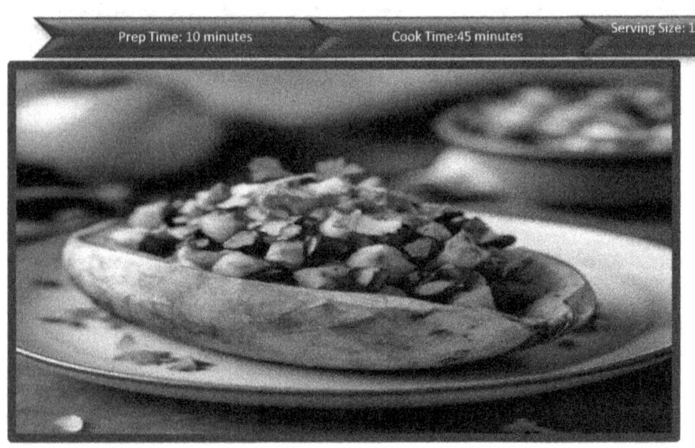

INGREDIENTS

Sweet potatoes, black beans, corn, red onion, bell pepper, lime juice, cilantro, cumin, olive oil, salt, pepper.

PREPARATION

Bake sweet potatoes until tender. Meanwhile, mix drained black beans, corn, diced red onion, diced bell pepper, lime juice, chopped cilantro, cumin, olive oil, salt, and pepper to make salsa. Serve sweet potatoes topped with black bean salsa.

Nutritional Information: High in fiber, protein, vitamins, and antioxidants.

Chapter 5:
Dinner Recipes

Baked Lemon Herb Chicken

Prep Time: 10 minutes | Cook Time: 25 minutes | Serving Size: 1 chicken breast.

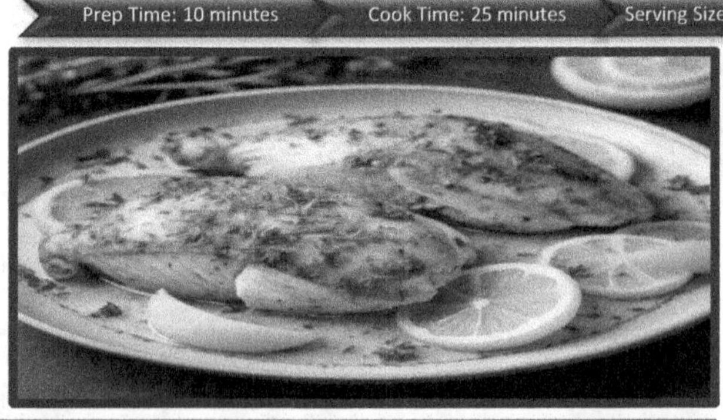

PREPARATION

Marinate chicken breasts with lemon juice, minced garlic, chopped thyme, rosemary, olive oil, salt, and pepper. Bake in the oven until cooked through.

INGREDIENTS

Chicken breasts, lemon, garlic, thyme, rosemary, olive oil, salt, pepper.

Nutritional Information: High in protein, vitamins, and minerals.

Roasted Salmon with Asparagus and Potatoes

Prep Time: 15 minutes | Cook Time: 25 minutes | 1 serving of salmon with vegetables.

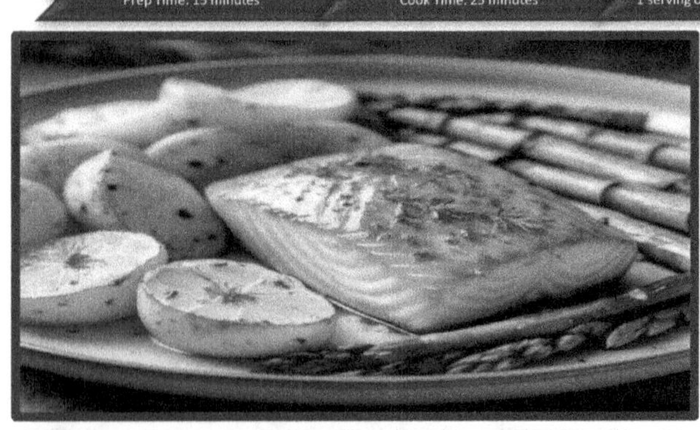

PREPARATION

Toss asparagus and potatoes with olive oil, garlic powder, lemon zest, salt, and pepper. Arrange on a baking sheet and place salmon fillets on top. Roast in the oven until salmon is cooked through and vegetables are tender.

INGREDIENTS

Salmon fillets, asparagus, potatoes, olive oil, garlic powder, lemon zest, salt, pepper.

Nutritional Information: High in omega-3 fatty acids, protein, fiber, and vitamins.

Turkey and Vegetable Stir-Fry

Prep Time: 10 minutes | Cook Time: 15 minutes | Serving Size: 1 serving of stir-fry with rice.

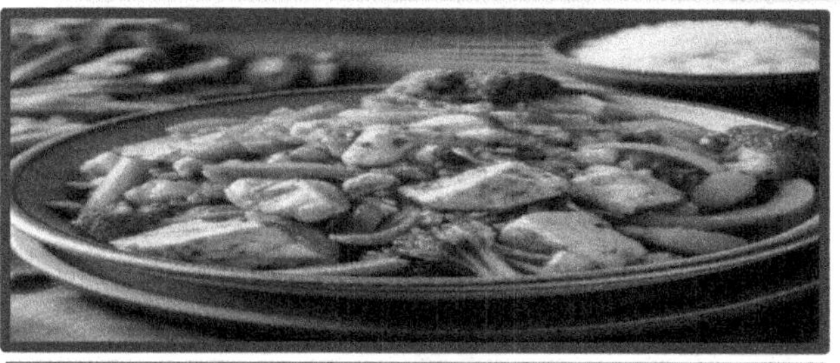

INGREDIENTS

Ground turkey, mixed vegetables (such as bell peppers, broccoli, snap peas), garlic, ginger, soy sauce, olive oil, brown rice.

PREPARATION

Cook ground turkey in olive oil until browned. Add minced garlic and ginger, then stir in mixed vegetables and soy sauce. Cook until vegetables are tender. Serve over cooked brown rice.

Nutritional Information: High in protein, fiber, vitamins, and minerals.

Quinoa and Black Bean Stuffed Zucchini Boats

Prep Time: 15 minutes | Cook Time: 25 minutes | Serving Size: 1 stuffed zucchini boat.

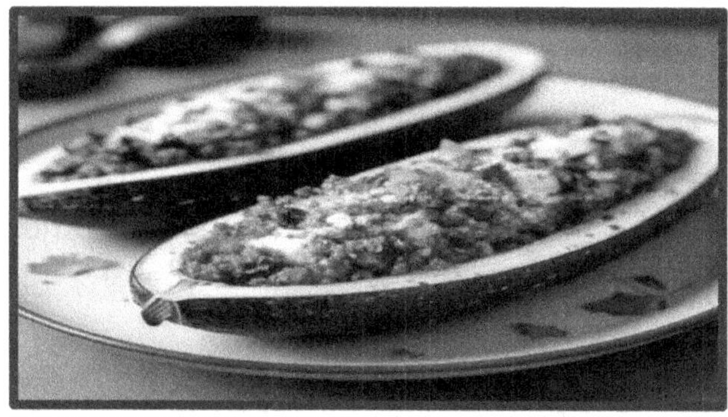

INGREDIENTS

Zucchini, quinoa, black beans, corn, onion, garlic, cumin, chili powder, salsa, shredded cheese (optional).

PREPARATION

Cut zucchini in half lengthwise and scoop out seeds to create "boats." Cook quinoa according to package instructions. Sauté onion and garlic until softened, then add cooked quinoa, black beans, corn, cumin, and chili powder. Stuff mixture into zucchini boats and bake until zucchini is tender. Serve with salsa and shredded cheese if desired.

Nutritional Information: High in protein, fiber, vitamins, and minerals.

Lentil and Vegetable Curry

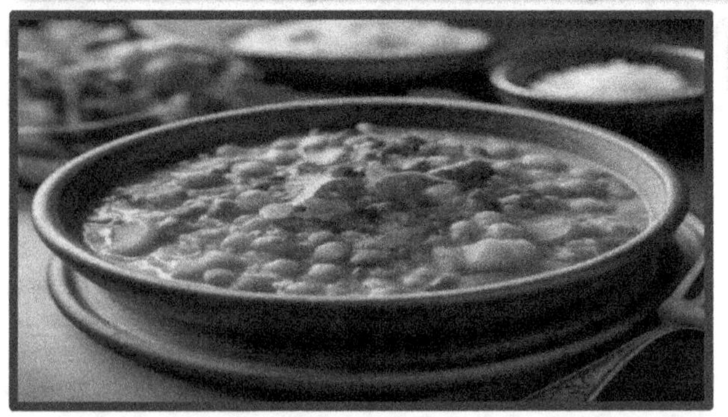

INGREDIENTS

Lentils, carrots, potatoes, onion, garlic, ginger, curry powder, coconut milk, vegetable broth, olive oil, salt, pepper.

PREPARATION

Sauté onion, garlic, and ginger in olive oil until fragrant. Add diced carrots and potatoes and cook until softened. Stir in cooked lentils, curry powder, coconut milk, and vegetable broth. Simmer until flavors meld together. Serve over cooked brown rice or quinoa.

Nutritional Information: High in protein, fiber, vitamins, and minerals.

Grilled Turkey Burgers with Sweet Potato Fries

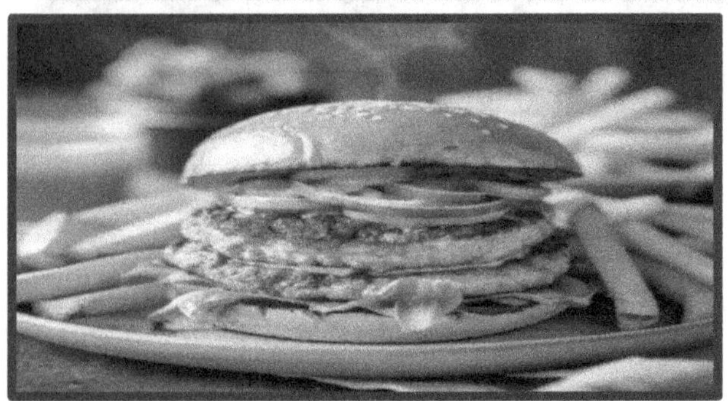

INGREDIENTS

Ground turkey, whole grain burger buns, lettuce, tomato, onion, sweet potatoes, olive oil, garlic powder, paprika, salt, pepper.

PREPARATION

Form ground turkey into patties and grill until cooked through. Slice sweet potatoes into fries, toss with olive oil, garlic powder, paprika, salt, and pepper, and bake until crispy. Serve turkey burgers on whole grain buns with lettuce, tomato, and onion, alongside sweet potato fries.

Nutritional Information: High in protein, fiber, vitamins, and minerals.

Mediterranean Chickpea Salad

Prep Time: 10 minutes | Cook Time: 0 minutes | Serving Size: 1 bowl of salad.

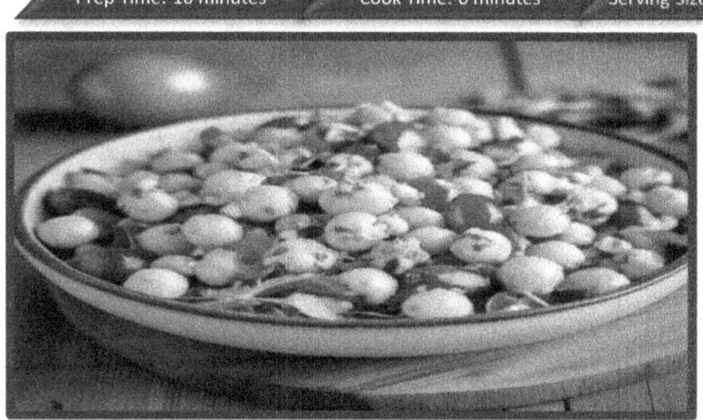

PREPARATION

Rinse and drain chickpeas. Dice cucumber, cherry tomatoes, red onion, and Kalamata olives. Crumble feta cheese and chop parsley. Toss together with lemon juice, olive oil, salt, and pepper.

INGREDIENTS

Chickpeas, cucumber, cherry tomatoes, red onion, Kalamata olives, feta cheese, parsley, lemon juice, olive oil, salt, pepper.

Nutritional Information: High in protein, fiber, healthy fats, and vitamins.

Eggplant Parmesan

Prep Time: 15 minutes | Cook Time 30 minutes | Serving Size: 1 serving of eggplant Parmesan

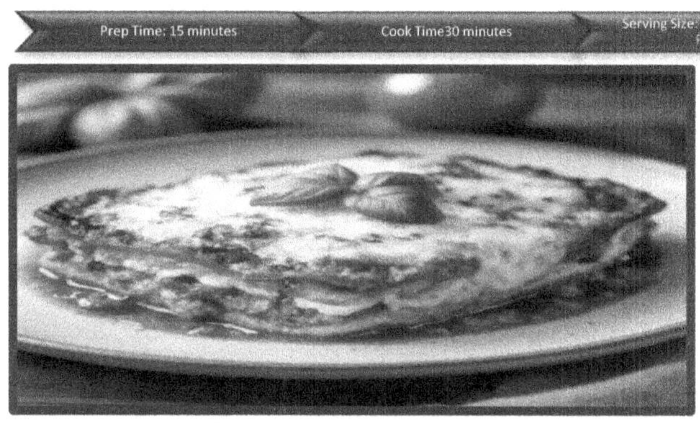

PREPARATION

Slice eggplant into rounds and dredge in whole wheat breadcrumbs mixed with grated Parmesan cheese. Bake until golden and crispy. Layer eggplant slices with marinara sauce and mozzarella cheese, then bake until cheese is melted and bubbly.

INGREDIENTS

Eggplant, whole wheat breadcrumbs, Parmesan cheese, marinara sauce, mozzarella cheese, olive oil, salt, pepper.

Nutritional Information: High in fiber, protein, vitamins, and minerals

Shrimp and Vegetable Skewers

Prep Time: 15minutes | Cook Time: 10 minutes | Serving Size: 1 serving of skewers.

INGREDIENTS

Shrimp, bell peppers, zucchini, cherry tomatoes, red onion, olive oil, garlic powder, lemon juice, salt, pepper.

PREPARATION

Thread shrimp and chopped vegetables onto skewers. Brush with olive oil, garlic powder, lemon juice, salt, and pepper. Grill until shrimp is cooked through and vegetables are tender.

Nutritional Information: High in protein, fiber, vitamins, and minerals.

Vegetable and Tofu Stir-Fry

Prep Time: 15minutes | Cook Time: 15 minutes | 1 serving of stir-fry with rice

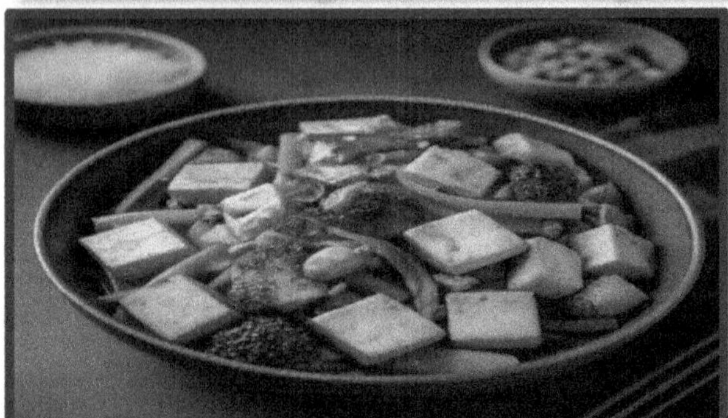

INGREDIENTS

Firm tofu, mixed vegetables (such as broccoli, bell peppers, snap peas), garlic, ginger, soy sauce, olive oil, brown rice.

PREPARATION

Press tofu to remove excess moisture, then cut into cubes. Sauté tofu in olive oil until golden. Add minced garlic and ginger, then stir in mixed vegetables and soy sauce. Cook until vegetables are tender. Serve over cooked brown rice.

Nutritional Information: High in protein, fiber, vitamins, and minerals

Chapter 6:
Snack Recipes

Greek Yogurt with Mixed Berries

Prep Time: 2minutes | Cook Time: 0 minutes | Serving Size: 1 bowl

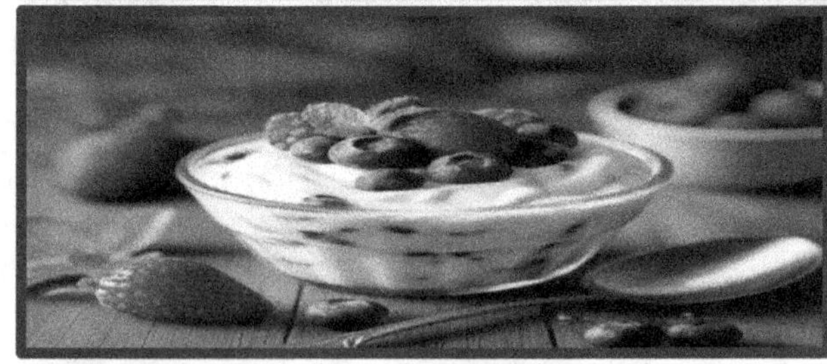

PREPARATION

Spoon Greek yogurt into a bowl and top with mixed berries. Drizzle with honey if desired.

INGREDIENTS

Greek yogurt, mixed berries (such as strawberries, blueberries, raspberries), honey (optional).

Nutritional Information: High in protein, probiotics, antioxidants, and vitamins.

Apple Slices with Almond Butter

INGREDIENTS

Apple, almond butter.

Prep Time: 5minutes | Cook Time0 minutes | Serving Size: 1 serving

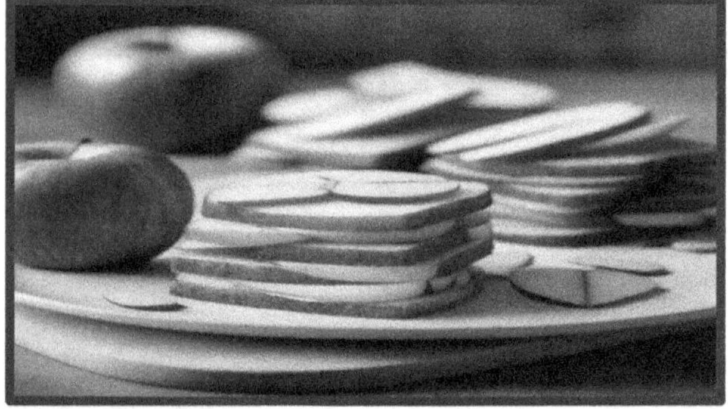

PREPARATION

Slice apple into wedges and serve with almond butter for dipping.

Nutritional Information: High in fiber, healthy fats, vitamins, and minerals.

Carrot Sticks with Hummus

INGREDIENTS

Carrot sticks, hummus.

Prep Time: 5 minutes   Cook Time: 0 minutes   Serving Size: 1 serving

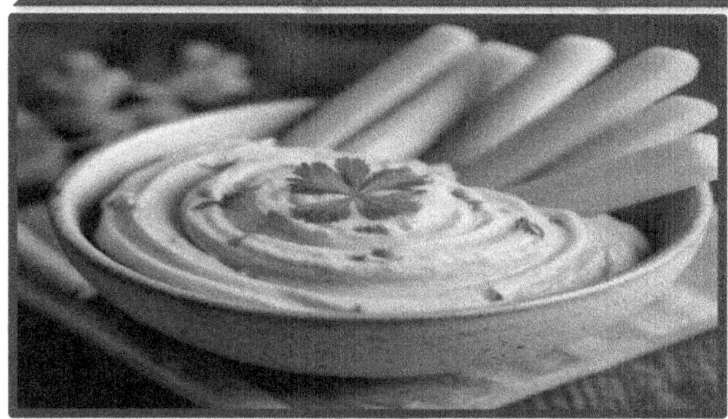

PREPARATION

Wash and peel carrots, then slice into sticks. Serve with hummus for dipping.

Nutritional Information: High in fiber, protein, vitamins, and minerals.

Rice Cake with Avocado

INGREDIENTS

Rice cake, avocado, salt, pepper, red pepper flakes (optional).

Prep Time: 2 minutes   Cook Time: 0 minutes   Serving Size: 1 rice cake.

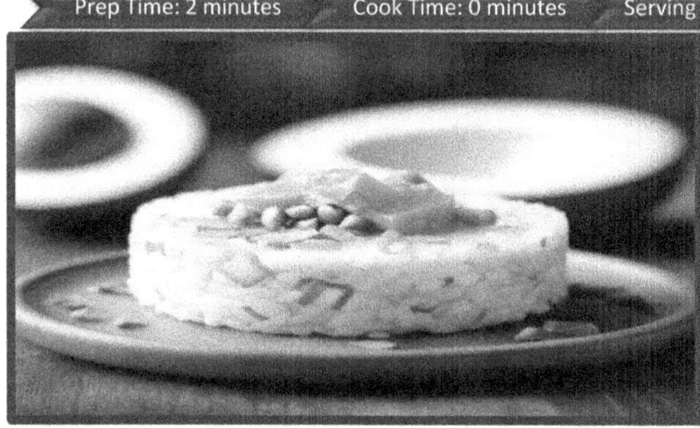

PREPARATION

Spread mashed avocado onto rice cake. Season with salt, pepper, and red pepper flakes if desired.

Nutritional Information: High in fiber, healthy fats, vitamins, and minerals.

Cottage Cheese with Pineapple

INGREDIENTS

Cottage cheese, pineapple chunks.

PREPARATION

Spoon cottage cheese into a bowl and top with pineapple chunks.

Nutritional Information: High in protein, calcium, vitamins, and minerals.
Prep Time: 2 minutes Cook Time: 0 minutes Serving Size: 1 serving.

Trail Mix with Nuts and Dried Fruit

Prep Time: 5minutes | Cook Time: 0 minutes | Serving Size: 1 serving.

INGREDIENTS

Almonds, walnuts, cashews, dried cranberries, dried apricots, dark chocolate chips.

Nutritional Information: High in protein, healthy fats, fiber, antioxidants, and vitamins.

PREPARATION

Mix together almonds, walnuts, cashews, dried cranberries, dried apricots, and dark chocolate chips.

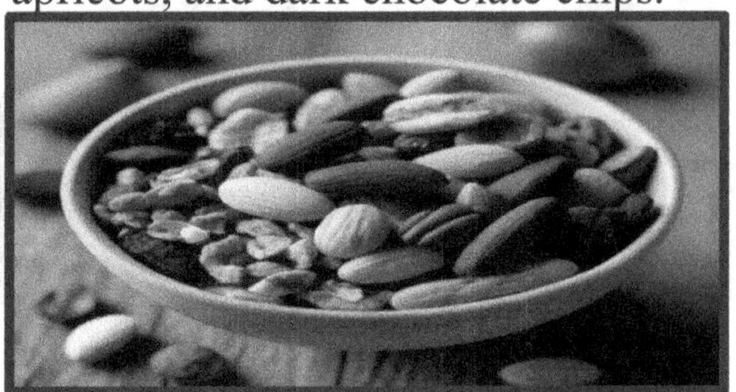

Veggie Sticks with Guacamole

INGREDIENTS

Carrot sticks, cucumber sticks, bell pepper strips, guacamole.

Prep Time: 5 minutes | Cook Time0minutes | Serving Size: 1 serving.

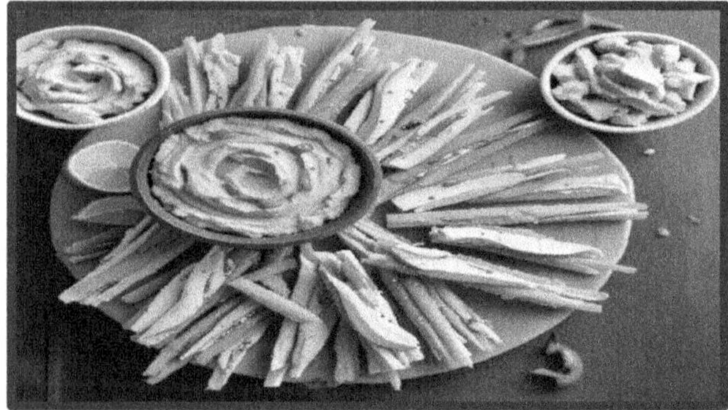

PREPARATION

Wash and cut vegetables into sticks and strips. Serve with guacamole for dipping.

Nutritional Information: High in fiber, healthy fats, vitamins, and minerals

Edamame Beans

INGREDIENT

Edamame beans (frozen or fresh), sea salt.

Prep Time: 5minutes | Cook Time: 5 minutes | Serving Size: 1 serving

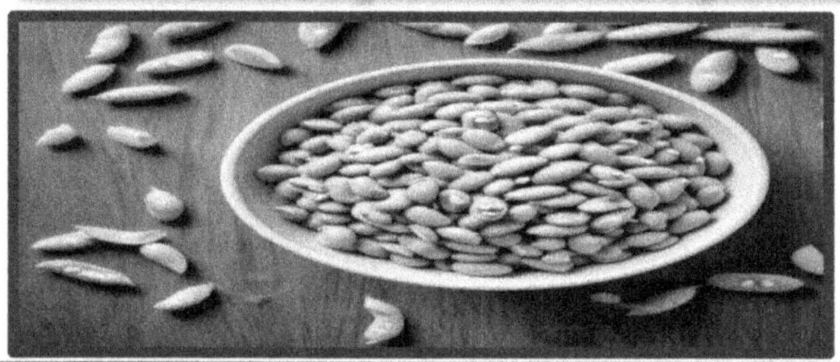

PREPARATION

Boil or steam edamame beans until tender. Sprinkle with sea salt before serving

Nutritional Information: High in protein, fiber, vitamins, and minerals.

Whole Grain Crackers with Tuna Salad

Prep Time: 5 minutes | Cook Time: 0 minutes | Serving Size: 1 serving.

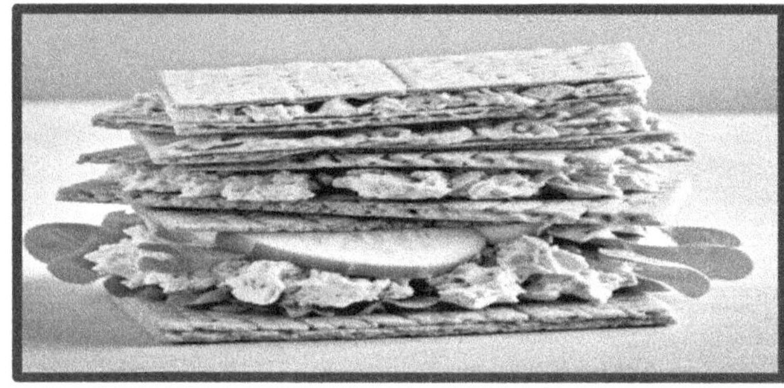

PREPARATION

Mix together drained canned tuna, Greek yogurt, diced celery, diced red onion, lemon juice, Dijon mustard, salt, and pepper. Serve tuna salad on top of whole grain crackers.

INGREDIENTS

Whole grain crackers, canned tuna, Greek yogurt, celery, red onion, lemon juice, Dijon mustard, salt, pepper.

Nutritional Information: High in protein, fiber, omega-3 fatty acids, vitamins, and minerals.

Cottage Cheese and Tomato Salad

Prep Time: 5 minutes
Cook Time: 0 minutes
Serving Size: 1 serving.

INGREDIENTS

Cottage cheese, cherry tomatoes, basil leaves, balsamic glaze (optional).

PREPARATION

Arrange cottage cheese, halved cherry tomatoes, and torn basil leaves on a plate. Drizzle with balsamic glaze if desired.

Nutritional Information: High in protein, calcium, vitamins, and minerals

Chapter 7:
Smoothies and
Drinks

Green Detox Smoothie

Prep Time: 5minutes | Cook Time: 0 minutes | Serving Size: 1 smoothie.

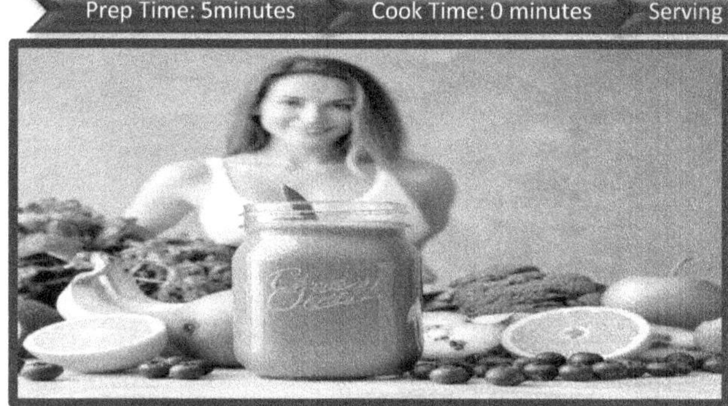

PREPARATION

Blend spinach, kale, cucumber, green apple, lemon juice, ginger, and water or coconut water until smooth. Add ice cubes and blend again until desired consistency is reached.

INGREDIENTS

Spinach, kale, cucumber, green apple, lemon juice, ginger, water or coconut water, ice cubes.

Nutritional Information: High in vitamins, minerals, antioxidants, and hydration.

Berry Blast Smoothie

Prep Time: 5minutes | Cook Time: 0 minutes | Serving Size: 1 smoothie.

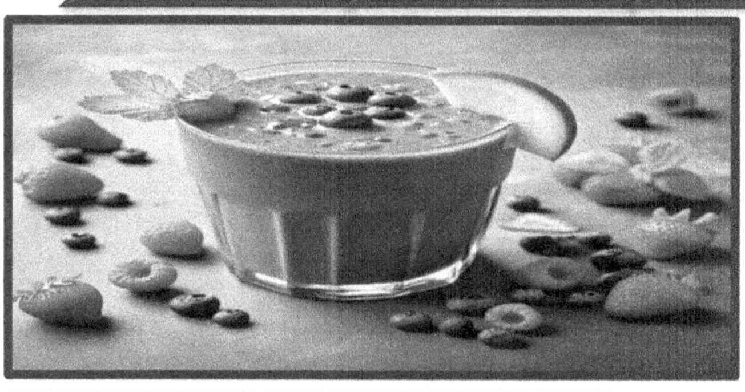

PREPARATION

Blend mixed berries, banana, Greek yogurt, almond milk, and honey until smooth. Add ice cubes and blend again until desired consistency is reached.

INGREDIENTS

Mixed berries (such as strawberries, blueberries, raspberries), banana, Greek yogurt, almond milk, honey (optional), ice cubes.

Nutritional Information: High in antioxidants, fiber, protein, and probiotics.

Tropical Turmeric Smoothie

Prep Time: 5 minutes   Cook Time: 0 minutes   Serving Size: 1 smoothie.

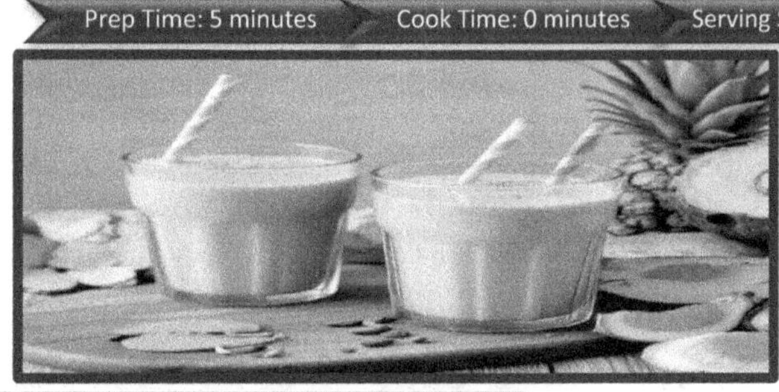

PREPARATION

Blend pineapple, mango, banana, coconut milk, turmeric, ginger, and honey until smooth. Add ice cubes and blend again until desired consistency is reached.

INGREDIENTS

Pineapple, mango, banana, coconut milk, turmeric, ginger, honey (optional), ice cubes.

Nutritional Information: High in vitamins, minerals, antioxidants, and anti-inflammatory compounds.

Avocado Banana Smoothie

Prep Time: 5 minutes   Cook Time: 0 minutes   Serving Size: 1 smoothie

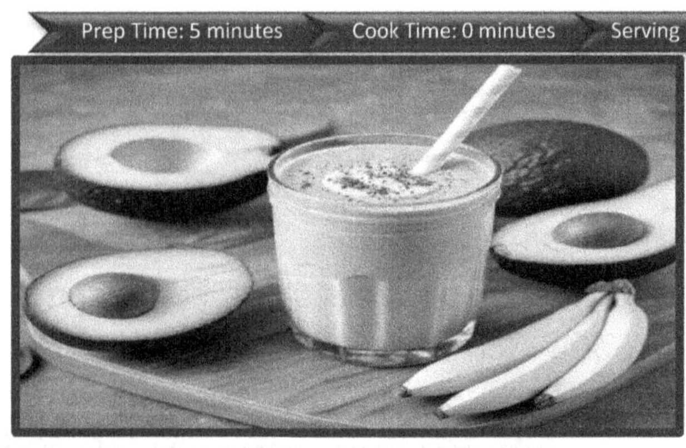

PREPARATION

Blend avocado, banana, spinach, almond milk, Greek yogurt, and honey until smooth. Add ice cubes and blend again until desired consistency is reached.

INGREDIENTS

Avocado, banana, spinach, almond milk, Greek yogurt, honey (optional), ice cubes.

Nutritional Information: High in healthy fats, fiber, vitamins, minerals, and probiotics.

Beetroot Berry Smoothie

Prep Time: 5 minutes   Cook Time: 0 minutes   Serving Size: 1 smoothie.

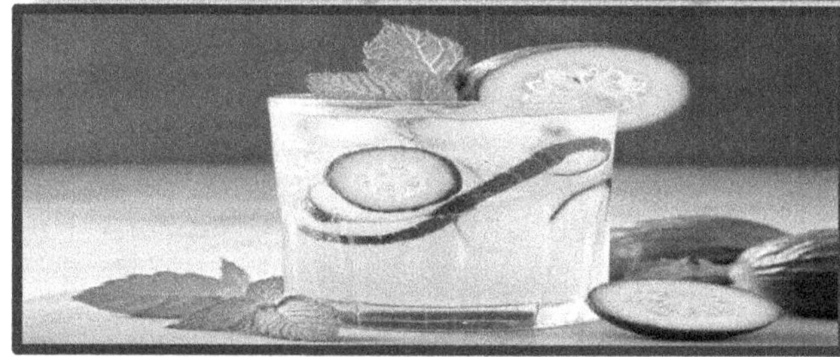

INGREDIENTS

Cooked beetroot, mixed berries (such as strawberries, blueberries, raspberries), Greek yogurt, almond milk, honey (optional), ice cubes.

PREPARATION

Blend cooked beetroot, mixed berries, Greek yogurt, almond milk, and honey until smooth. Add ice cubes and blend again until desired consistency is reached.

Nutritional Information: High in antioxidants, fiber, vitamins, minerals, and probiotics.

Cucumber Mint Cooler

Prep Time: 5 minutes   Cook Time: 0 minutes   Serving Size: 1 glass.

PREPARATION

Blend cucumber, mint leaves, lime juice, honey, and water until smooth. Add ice cubes and blend again until desired consistency is reached.

INGREDIENTS

Cucumber, mint leaves, lime juice, honey (optional), water, ice cubes.

Nutritional Information: High in hydration, vitamins, minerals, and antioxidants.

Golden Milk Latte

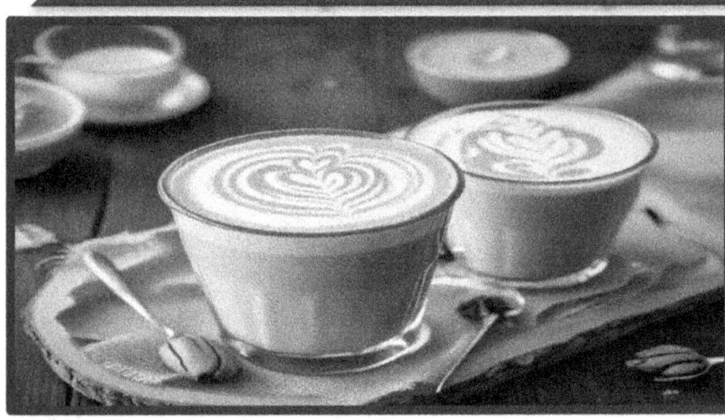

INGREDIENTS

Almond milk, turmeric, cinnamon, ginger, honey (optional).

PREPARATION

Warm almond milk in a saucepan over low heat. Stir in turmeric, cinnamon, ginger, and honey until well combined. Pour into a mug and serve warm.

Nutritional Information: High in anti-inflammatory compounds, vitamins, minerals, and antioxidants.

Citrus Green Tea

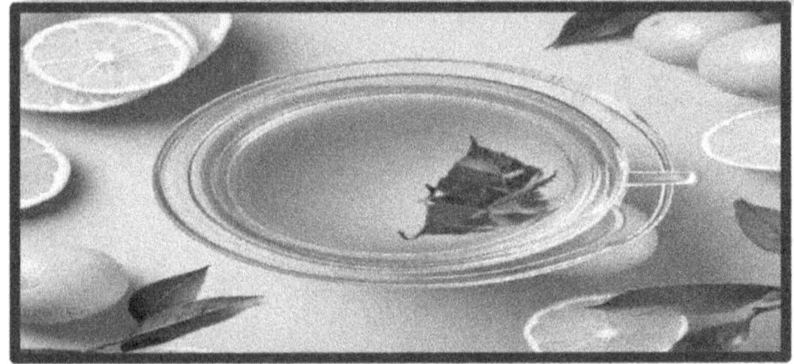

PREPARATION

Brew green tea and let it cool to room temperature. Add lemon slices, lime slices, orange slices, and honey to the tea. Serve over ice.

INGREDIENTS

Green tea, lemon slices, lime slices, orange slices, honey (optional), ice cubes.

Nutritional Information: High in antioxidants, vitamins, and hydration.

Watermelon Mint Refresher

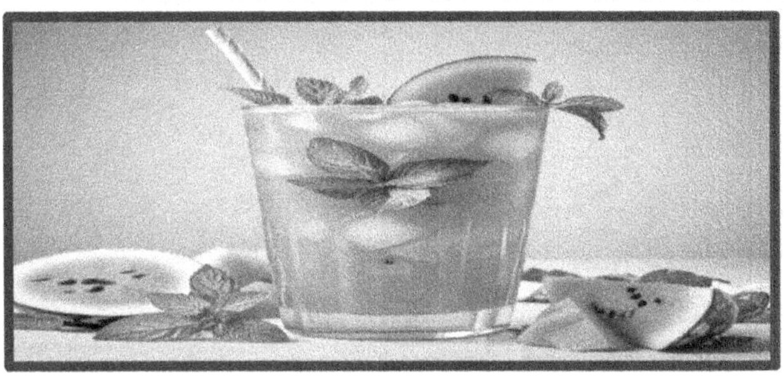

INGREDIENTS

Watermelon, mint leaves, lime juice, honey (optional), water, ice cubes.

PREPARATION

Blend watermelon, mint leaves, lime juice, honey, and water until smooth. Add ice cubes and blend again until desired consistency is reached.

Nutritional Information: High in hydration, vitamins, minerals, and antioxidants.

Peach Ginger Iced Tea

INGREDIENTS

Peach slices, ginger slices, black tea bags, water, honey (optional), ice cubes.

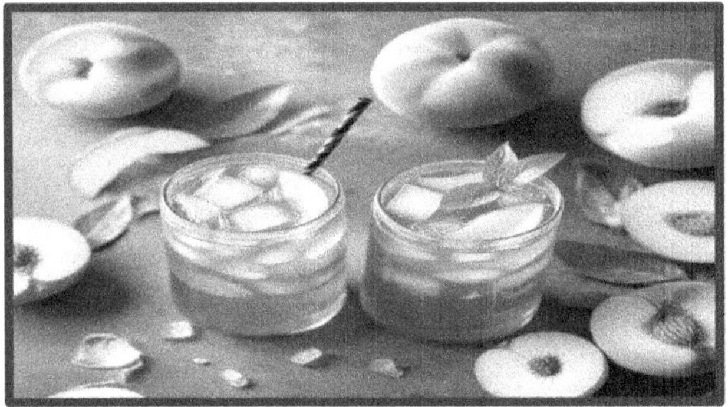

PREPARATION

Steep black tea bags in hot water with peach slices and ginger slices. Let it cool to room temperature, then refrigerate until chilled. Serve over ice with honey if desired.

Nutritional Information: High in antioxidants, vitamins, minerals, and hydration.

Chapter 8

Useful Bonus: Tips for Managing Fatty Liver Disease

Staying hydrated is a fundamental aspect of overall health and wellness, particularly for those managing conditions such as fatty liver disease. Adequate hydration supports numerous bodily functions, including liver function, digestion, and metabolic processes. Here's an in-depth look at the importance of hydration and how to ensure you stay properly hydrated:

The Importance of Hydration

1. Supports Liver Function: The liver plays a crucial role in detoxifying the body by filtering toxins and waste products from the blood. Adequate hydration helps the liver perform these functions more efficiently by maintaining optimal blood flow and enabling the proper elimination of toxins through urine.

2. Aids Digestion and Nutrient Absorption: Water is essential for the digestion of food and the absorption of nutrients. It helps break down food in the stomach and intestines, making nutrients available for absorption into the bloodstream.

3. Regulates Body Temperature: Water is vital for regulating body temperature through sweating and respiration. Staying hydrated ensures that your body can cool itself effectively, especially during exercise or in hot weather.

4. Enhances Metabolic Function: Hydration is key to maintaining an efficient metabolism. Water is involved in almost every metabolic process in the body, including the breakdown of fats and carbohydrates for energy.

5. Promotes Healthy Skin: Proper hydration keeps your skin moisturized and can improve its elasticity and appearance. Dehydration can lead to dry, flaky skin and exacerbate skin conditions.

6. Improves Cognitive Function: Dehydration can impair cognitive functions such as concentration, memory, and alertness. Staying hydrated supports brain function and mental clarity.

7. Prevents Constipation: Water helps soften stool and promotes regular bowel movements, preventing constipation and promoting overall digestive health.

How to Stay Hydrated

1. Drink Plenty of Water: Aim to drink at least 8 glasses (about 2 liters) of water per day. Individual needs may vary based on factors such as age, activity level, and climate.

2. Monitor Your Hydration: A simple way to monitor your hydration status is by checking the color of your urine. Pale yellow urine typically indicates good hydration, while dark yellow or amber urine may suggest dehydration.

3. Include Hydrating Foods: Incorporate foods with high water content into your diet, such as:

- Fruits: Watermelon, oranges, strawberries, and cucumbers.
- Vegetables: Lettuce, celery, tomatoes, and zucchini.

4. Limit Dehydrating Beverages: Reduce consumption of beverages that can dehydrate you, such as those high in caffeine (coffee, certain teas, energy drinks) and alcohol. If consumed, balance them with additional water intake.

5. Start Your Day with Water: Begin your day by drinking a glass of water to kickstart your hydration. This can also help wake up your metabolism and digestive system.

6. Carry a Water Bottle: Keep a reusable water bottle with you throughout the day to encourage regular water consumption. Sip on water regularly, even if you don't feel thirsty.

7. Set Hydration Goals: Set daily hydration goals and track your water intake. There are various apps and tools available that can help you stay on track with your hydration needs.

8. Flavor Your Water: If plain water doesn't appeal to you, try adding natural flavorings such as lemon, lime, mint, or berries to make it more enjoyable.

9. Drink Water Before Meals: Drinking a glass of water before meals can help with digestion and prevent overeating by creating a sense of fullness.

10. Stay Hydrated During Exercise: Ensure you drink water before, during, and after physical activity to replace fluids lost through sweat and maintain performance.

Limiting Alcohol Intake

Drinking alcohol has a big impact on liver health, particularly for those who have fatty liver disease or are at risk for it. Alcohol may worsen liver disease and impair the liver's capacity to function. Here is a detailed explanation of the importance of reducing alcohol use, as well as achievable methods to do so:

Alcohol's effects on liver health

1. Liver Damage: Drinking too much alcohol may damage the liver and cause cirrhosis, alcoholic hepatitis, and alcoholic fatty liver disease (AFLD). Large quantities of alcohol are too much for the liver to handle and cleanse, which causes inflammation, scarring, and decreased liver function.

2. Alcohol may exacerbate liver damage in those who have non-alcoholic fatty liver disease (NAFLD). Simple fatty liver disease may progress more quickly to more serious disorders, including non-alcoholic steatohepatitis (NASH) and fibrosis, even with modest drinking.

3. Interference with Metabolism: Alcohol interferes with the way that fats and carbohydrates are normally metabolized, which leads to the buildup of fat in the liver. This may lead to insulin resistance and other metabolic abnormalities, exacerbating fatty liver disease.

4. Increased Oxidative Stress: The alcohol metabolism produces toxic byproducts that make the liver more vulnerable to oxidative stress. In addition to harming liver cells, this stress promotes fibrosis and inflammation.

Benefits of Reducing Alcohol Consumption

1. Lessened liver stress: Reducing alcohol use eases the strain on your liver and promotes better recovery and function. This is essential to stopping liver disease from becoming worse.

2. Better General Health: Cutting down on alcohol may help with weight control, better digestion, better sleep, and increased mental clarity, among other health benefits.

3. Reduced chance of liver cancer: Long-term alcohol use raises the chance of developing liver cancer. You can greatly lower this risk by consuming less alcohol.

4. Improved Blood Sugar Control: Alcohol may impact insulin sensitivity and blood sugar levels. Restricting consumption may aid in keeping blood sugar levels steady, which is crucial for those who have diabetes or are at risk of developing it.

Effective Techniques to Reduce Alcohol Consumption

1. Establish Specific Objectives: Establish clear, attainable objectives, and decide why you are restricting your alcohol intake. Setting specific goals will help you remain on track, whether that goal is to cut down on beverages or stop entirely.

2. Monitor Consumption: Count the amount of alcohol you drink. Track your alcohol consumption using a notebook or an app to spot trends that should be altered.

3. Choose Alcohol-Free Days: Set aside certain days of the week for non-alcoholic periods. The number of these days should be increased gradually as you become used to cutting down on your consumption.

4. Select Non-Alcoholic Substitutes: Savor non-alcoholic drinks like mocktails, herbal teas, and sparkling water. When lounging or mingling, they might be fulfilling substitutes.

5. Be Aware of Social Circumstances: Make advance plans for social gatherings where alcohol will be served. If you intend to consume any alcohol at all, make a decision in advance and follow through on it. To get their support, share your goals with loved ones.

6. Cope with peer pressure: Acquire the skill of graciously refusing alcohol offers. Prepare a retort, such as "I'm cutting back on alcohol" or "I'm focusing on my health."

7. Take Up New Activities: Look for new pastimes and pastimes that don't include drinking. You may divert your attention from drinking by engaging in hobbies like reading, writing, art projects, or clubbing.

8. Seek Support: Participate in online forums or support groups where you may talk about your experiences and get motivation from those who are also reducing their alcohol use.

9. Educate yourself: Learn about the physiological effects of alcohol and the benefits of consuming less of it. This information may strengthen your resolve to make savings.

10. Professional Assistance: Consult a counselor or medical professional with expertise in addiction and drug misuse if you are unable to reduce your alcohol intake on your own.

Reducing alcohol use is essential for preserving liver health, particularly for those who are treating fatty liver disease. Understanding how alcohol affects the liver and implementing doable measures to cut down on drinking might help you stay much healthier overall and stop liver disease from becoming worse. Adopt a more health-conscious way of living and cut down on alcohol to help your liver mend and improve your overall wellbeing.

Monitoring Sugar Intake

Consuming too much sugar may be harmful to one's general health, especially for those who are coping with fatty liver disease. It's critical to keep an eye on sugar consumption and cut down if you want to improve liver function, stop more problems, and feel better overall. Here's a detailed look at the importance of controlling sugar consumption and doable ways to do so:

Sugar's Effect on Liver Health

1. Encourages Fat Accumulation: Fructose, a form of sugar that is included in a lot of sweetened foods and drinks, may cause the liver to produce more fat when consumed in excess. This encourages the buildup of liver fat, which worsens fatty liver disease.

2. Increases Insulin Resistance: Consuming a lot of sugar may exacerbate insulin resistance, a disorder in which the body's cells are unable to react to insulin as they should. Non-alcoholic fatty liver disease (NAFLD) development and progression are directly associated with insulin resistance.

3. Triggers Inflammation: Sugar has the ability to cause inflammation in the liver as well as other parts of the body. Prolonged inflammation has the potential to harm the liver and raise the possibility of developing more serious liver diseases, including non-alcoholic steatohepatitis (NASH).

4. Contributes to Obesity: Consuming a lot of sugar has a big impact on weight gain and obesity. Obesity is one of the leading risk factors for metabolic diseases, such as fatty liver disease.

5. Impacts on Overall Metabolic Health: Consuming too much sugar may interfere with regular metabolic functions, raising the risk of type 2 diabetes, cardiovascular disease, and other illnesses.

Benefits of Monitoring Sugar Intake:

1. Reduces Liver Fat: Reducing your intake of sugar, especially fructose, can help you manage and improve fatty liver disease by lowering the amount of fat that is created and stored in your liver.

2. Enhances Insulin Sensitivity: Cutting down on sugar helps improve insulin sensitivity, which lowers the risk of type 2 diabetes and helps to control blood sugar levels.

3. Reduces Inflammation: Cutting down on sugar intake may help the body's inflammatory response, which improves general health and eases the strain on the liver.

4. Promotes Weight Management: Sugar monitoring and restriction may assist with weight reduction and maintenance of a healthy weight, which is advantageous for general health and liver function.

5. Boosts Energy Levels: Reducing sugar intake helps maintain energy levels and avoid the crashes and spikes that come with consuming large amounts of sugar.

Effective Techniques for Tracking and Reducing Sugar Consumption

1. Examine food labels: Learn how to read labels. Look for added sugars in the nutritional information on food packages. High-fructose corn syrup, sucrose, glucose, and other sweets are ingredients to be wary of.

2. Select Natural Sweeteners: In moderation, use natural sweeteners like honey or maple syrup. Compared to refined sugar, they are less processed and could provide some nutritional advantages.

3. Limit Sugary Drinks: Cut down on soda, fruit juices, and other beverages with added sugar. These drinks have a substantial amount of added sugar. Opt instead for unsweetened drinks, herbal teas, or water.

4. Consume Whole Foods: Give priority to unprocessed, whole foods such as fruits, vegetables, whole grains, lean meats, and healthy fats. These foods provide vital nutrients and are naturally low in sugar.

5. Be Aware of Hidden Sugars: Take note of hidden sugars in meals like bread, dressings, sauces, and processed snacks that may not taste sweet. Choose handmade versions so you can be in charge of the ingredients.

6. Use sugar substitutes: Stevia and erythritol are two sugar alternatives that deliver sweetness without having the same effect on blood sugar levels. Use them sparingly, however, and be aware of any possible intestinal problems.

7. Fulfill Your Need for Sweets Healthy tip: Pick fruit if you're seeking something sweet. In addition to satisfying your sweet craving, berries, apples, and pears also provide fiber and other minerals.

8. Cook at Home: When you cook at home, you can regulate how much sugar is in your food. Try reducing the sugar in recipes and looking for healthier substitutes.

9. Make Reasonable Goals: Gradually reduce sugar so that your taste receptors can get used to it. Start by reducing the amount of sugar you put in your tea or coffee, as well as the amount of sweet foods you consume.

10. Seek support: To properly monitor and reduce your sugar consumption, join support groups or see a nutritionist or dietitian.

The purpose of treating fatty liver disease and improving general health, sugar consumption must be closely monitored and reduced. Consuming too much sugar may worsen the buildup of liver fat, raise insulin resistance, and fuel obesity and inflammation. You can drastically cut down on sugar by implementing sensible habits such as reading food labels, choosing natural sweeteners, avoiding sugar-filled drinks, and emphasizing whole meals. Your general health will be improved, your metabolic function will be enhanced, and your liver health will be supported by these improvements.

Choosing Healthy Fats

Choosing the appropriate fats is essential for preserving general health, especially for those who are treating fatty liver disease. While harmful fats may worsen liver problems and cause other chronic illnesses, good fats can support liver function, lower inflammation, and improve heart health. Here's a detailed examination of the significance of selecting healthful fats and doable methods for include them in your diet:

The Value of Healthful Fats

1. Promotes Liver Health: Unsaturated fats in particular may help lower liver fat and enhance liver function. They also aid in the absorption of fat-soluble vitamins, which are essential for good health generally and include A, D, E, and K.

2. Reduces Inflammation: The anti-inflammatory characteristics of healthy fats, especially omega-3 fatty acids, may aid in reducing inflammation in the liver and other areas of the body.

3. Encourages Heart Health: The risk of heart disease may be decreased by consuming unsaturated fats, such as monounsaturated and polyunsaturated fats, which can help boost HDL (good cholesterol) and reduce LDL (bad cholesterol).

4. Improves Metabolic Function: Hormone synthesis, the integrity of cell membranes, and energy balance are just a few of the metabolic activities that healthy fats are essential for sustaining.

5. Offers Satiety: Due to their higher calorie density compared to proteins and carbs, fats give off a satiety that may help control hunger and stop overindulging.

Different Types of Healthful Fats

1. Fats Not Saturated:
Found in: seeds, avocados, almonds, cashews, and peanuts; nuts.
Benefits: Offers antioxidant qualities, lowers bad cholesterol, and promotes cardiovascular health in general.

2. Fats Polyunsaturated:
Found in: Walnuts, flaxseeds, chia seeds, sunflower oil, and fatty fish (salmon, mackerel, and sardines).
Benefits: Contains omega-3 and omega-6 fatty acids, which are critical for cell development, inflammation reduction, and brain function.
3. Fatty Acids Omega-3:
Found in: Leafy green vegetables, walnuts, chia seeds, flaxseed oil, and fish oil
Benefits: May enhance liver fat metabolism, lower inflammation, and promote heart health.
4. Fatty Acids Omega-6:
Found in: Nuts, soybean oil, safflower oil, and sunflower oil.
Benefits: Necessary for healthy brain development and growth. It's critical to maintain an omega-3 balance to prevent aggravating inflammation.

Types of Fats That Are Not Good for You

1. Trans Fats:
Found in: Margarine, baked items, fried foods, and processed foods.
Risks: boosts the risk of heart disease, stroke, and type 2 diabetes. Lowers good cholesterol (HDL) and boosts bad cholesterol (LDL).
2. Fats That Are Saturated:
Found in: Full-fat dairy products, butter, cheese, and red meat.
Risks: When ingested in excess, it elevate bad cholesterol levels and increase the risk of heart disease.

Realistic Techniques for Including Healthy Fats

1. Cook with Healthful Oils: Instead of using butter or lard, use oils high in monounsaturated and polyunsaturated fats, including canola or olive oil.
2. Eat Fatty Fish: To increase your intake of omega-3 fatty acids, include fatty fish like salmon, mackerel, and sardines in your diet at least twice a week.
3. Snack on Nuts and Seeds: As a nutritious snack, go for nuts and seeds. They are a wonderful supply of protein, fiber, and healthy fats. For best results, use raw or unsalted types.

4. Add Avocados: Use avocados in smoothies, salads, and sandwiches. They provide vital nutrients like fiber and potassium and are high in monounsaturated fats.

5. Use Chia and Flaxseeds: Include chia or flaxseeds in porridge, smoothies, and yogurt. They are great providers of fiber and omega-3 fatty acids.

6. Read Labels: Consult food labels to minimize saturated fats and stay away from trans fats. Seek for goods with less processed components and better fat profiles.

7. Opt for Lean Proteins: To lower your consumption of saturated fat, choose lean protein sources like fish, chicken, beans, and lentils rather than red meat.

8. Limit Processed meals: Because processed and fried meals are often heavy in bad fats, cut down on your intake of them. Make meals at home using complete, fresh ingredients.

9. Omega-6 and Omega-3 Balance: Make sure your intake of these two fatty acids is equal. Increase your intake of foods high in omega-3 fatty acids since the average Western diet is generally heavy in omega-6 and low in omega-3.

10. Use Nut Butters: For spreads or additions to smoothies and snacks, use natural nut butters (free of hydrogenated fats or added sugars).

Selecting healthful fats is crucial for boosting heart health, lowering inflammation, maintaining liver function, and improving general wellbeing. You may improve your health by include sources of monounsaturated and polyunsaturated fats, especially omega-3 fatty acids, and avoiding trans and excessively saturated fats. Use these useful tips to maintain a nutritious, well-balanced diet and get the advantages of healthy fats.

Conclusion

Developing a regimented eating plan has several benefits, particularly when trying to control and enhance diseases like fatty liver disease. Here are some of the main advantages:

1. Equilibrium Nutrition

Assures Sufficient Nutrient Intake: Following a planned meal plan makes it more likely that you'll eat a healthy, well-balanced diet full of vital nutrients. This equilibrium is critical for both sustained liver function and overall health.

Prevents Nutrient Shortages: Common nutrient shortages may be avoided by adhering to a food plan. A range of foods are included in the diet to provide vitamins, minerals, proteins, healthy fats, and carbs.

2. Promotes hepatic function

Reduces Liver Fat: A structured meal plan for fatty liver disease aims to reduce liver fat by including foods that are rich in fiber, antioxidants, and healthy fats, as well as low in saturated fats.

Encourages Liver Detoxification: The diet includes items that help the liver's natural detoxification activities, such as almonds, citrus fruits, and leafy greens.

3. Promotes healthy weight management

A structured meal plan may help with weight loss by offering portion-controlled, calorie-conscious meals that discourage overeating and encourage a healthy weight.

Maintains a Healthy Weight: By guaranteeing a balanced calorie intake, a meal plan assists those who do not need to lose weight in maintaining a healthy weight.

4. Makes meal preparation simpler

Saves Time: By offering a clear direction on what to eat and when, an organized meal plan makes meal preparation simpler. This cuts down on the amount of time spent grocery shopping and meal planning.

Promotes Batch Cooking: Preparing meals in advance enables batch cooking, which may save time and ease the strain of everyday cooking.

5. Enhances Eating Patterns

Cuts Down on Bad Decisions: When you have a strategy in place, you are less likely to make rash and unwise dietary decisions. This makes it easier to maintain a balanced diet over time.

Encourages Consistent Eating Patterns: Regular meal times are encouraged by structured eating schedules, which may enhance digestion and metabolism in general.

6. Increases appreciation and variety of food

Introducing new dishes: Adding diversity to your diet and avoiding meal monotony, a meal plan promotes experimenting with new dishes and ingredients.

Enhances Relationships with Food: Eating may be a more joyful and attentive experience when you approach meals with a positive and organized mindset.

7. Encourages general health.

Boosts Energy Levels: Eating meals that are well-balanced and nutrient-rich will greatly increase your energy levels and general vigor.

Improves Mental Well-Being: There is a direct correlation between mental health and proper diet. A well-organized meal plan may improve mood and cognitive performance, while also easing the tension and worry associated with meal preparation.

8. Makes it easier to monitor nutrition and health

Simpler Monitoring and Tracking for Healthcare Professionals: When healthcare practitioners adhere to a planned strategy, they may be able to monitor and track patients more easily. Based on a regular eating pattern, they may provide more knowledgeable advice and modifications.

Aids in the Identification of Food Sensitivities: By methodically removing and reintroducing foods, an organized method may assist in the identification of any food sensitivities or allergies.

9. Economical

Reduces food loss: You may save money on wasted or ruined food by organizing your meals and grocery shopping in a way that minimizes food loss.

Promotes Cost-Effective Decisions: A meal plan encourages buying just what is required, which often results in more frugal decisions and the avoidance of wasteful spending.

There are several advantages to following a planned diet, especially for those with fatty liver disease. It guarantees nutritional balance, promotes liver health, helps control weight, makes meal preparation easier, strengthens dietary habits, increases food variety and pleasure, promotes general health, makes medical monitoring easier, and is reasonably priced. You can take charge of your diet, improve your health, and enjoy preparing tasty, healthy meals for your body by adhering to a set schedule.

Acknowledgments

I would like to express my heartfelt gratitude to the following individuals for their invaluable support and contributions to this book:

- My family, for their unwavering encouragement and belief in my endeavors.
- My friends, for their inspiration and enthusiasm throughout this journey.
- The dedicated team at the publishing house, for their expertise and guidance in bringing this book to fruition.
- The readers, whose curiosity and passion for health and wellness continue to inspire me every day.

Thank you for being a part of this journey.

WEEKLY MEAL PLANNING

Month: _______________

Week:

(1) (2) (3) (4)

Sunday

Breakfast: _______________

Calories	Protein	Sugar	Carbs

Lunch: _______________

Calories	Protein	Sugar	Carbs

Dinner: _______________

Calories	Protein	Sugar	Carbs

Monday

Breakfast: _______________

Calories	Protein	Sugar	Carbs

Lunch: _______________

Calories	Protein	Sugar	Carbs

Dinner: _______________

Calories	Protein	Sugar	Carbs

Tuesday

Breakfast: _______________

Calories	Protein	Sugar	Carbs

Lunch: _______________

Calories	Protein	Sugar	Carbs

Dinner: _______________

Calories	Protein	Sugar	Carbs

Wednesday

Breakfast: _______________

Calories	Protein	Sugar	Carbs

Lunch: _______________

Calories	Protein	Sugar	Carbs

Dinner: _______________

Calories	Protein	Sugar	Carbs

Thursday

Breakfast: _______________

Calories	Protein	Sugar	Carbs

Lunch: _______________

Calories	Protein	Sugar	Carbs

Dinner: _______________

Calories	Protein	Sugar	Carbs

Friday

Breakfast: _______________

Calories	Protein	Sugar	Carbs

Lunch: _______________

Calories	Protein	Sugar	Carbs

Dinner: _______________

Calories	Protein	Sugar	Carbs

Saturday

Breakfast: _______________

Calories	Protein	Sugar	Carbs

Lunch: _______________

Calories	Protein	Sugar	Carbs

Dinner: _______________

Calories	Protein	Sugar	Carbs

Shopping List:

WEEKLY MEAL PLANNING

Month: ______________

Week:

(1) (2) (3) (4)

Sunday

Breakfast: ______________

Calories	Protein	Sugar	Carbs

Lunch: ______________

Calories	Protein	Sugar	Carbs

Dinner: ______________

Calories	Protein	Sugar	Carbs

Monday

Breakfast: ______________

Calories	Protein	Sugar	Carbs

Lunch: ______________

Calories	Protein	Sugar	Carbs

Dinner: ______________

Calories	Protein	Sugar	Carbs

Tuesday

Breakfast: ______________

Calories	Protein	Sugar	Carbs

Lunch: ______________

Calories	Protein	Sugar	Carbs

Dinner: ______________

Calories	Protein	Sugar	Carbs

Wednesday

Breakfast: ______________

Calories	Protein	Sugar	Carbs

Lunch: ______________

Calories	Protein	Sugar	Carbs

Dinner: ______________

Calories	Protein	Sugar	Carbs

Thursday

Breakfast: ______________

Calories	Protein	Sugar	Carbs

Lunch: ______________

Calories	Protein	Sugar	Carbs

Dinner: ______________

Calories	Protein	Sugar	Carbs

Friday

Breakfast: ______________

Calories	Protein	Sugar	Carbs

Lunch: ______________

Calories	Protein	Sugar	Carbs

Dinner: ______________

Calories	Protein	Sugar	Carbs

Saturday

Breakfast: ______________

Calories	Protein	Sugar	Carbs

Lunch: ______________

Calories	Protein	Sugar	Carbs

Dinner: ______________

Calories	Protein	Sugar	Carbs

Shopping List:

WEEKLY MEAL PLANNING

Month: ___________________

Week:

(1) (2) (3) (4)

Sunday

Breakfast: ___________________

Calories	Protein	Sugar	Carbs

Lunch: ___________________

Calories	Protein	Sugar	Carbs

Dinner: ___________________

Calories	Protein	Sugar	Carbs

Monday

Breakfast: ___________________

Calories	Protein	Sugar	Carbs

Lunch: ___________________

Calories	Protein	Sugar	Carbs

Dinner: ___________________

Calories	Protein	Sugar	Carbs

Tuesday

Breakfast: ___________________

Calories	Protein	Sugar	Carbs

Lunch: ___________________

Calories	Protein	Sugar	Carbs

Dinner: ___________________

Calories	Protein	Sugar	Carbs

Wednesday

Breakfast: ___________________

Calories	Protein	Sugar	Carbs

Lunch: ___________________

Calories	Protein	Sugar	Carbs

Dinner: ___________________

Calories	Protein	Sugar	Carbs

Thursday

Breakfast: ___________________

Calories	Protein	Sugar	Carbs

Lunch: ___________________

Calories	Protein	Sugar	Carbs

Dinner: ___________________

Calories	Protein	Sugar	Carbs

Friday

Breakfast: ___________________

Calories	Protein	Sugar	Carbs

Lunch: ___________________

Calories	Protein	Sugar	Carbs

Dinner: ___________________

Calories	Protein	Sugar	Carbs

Saturday

Breakfast: ___________________

Calories	Protein	Sugar	Carbs

Lunch: ___________________

Calories	Protein	Sugar	Carbs

Dinner: ___________________

Calories	Protein	Sugar	Carbs

Shopping List:

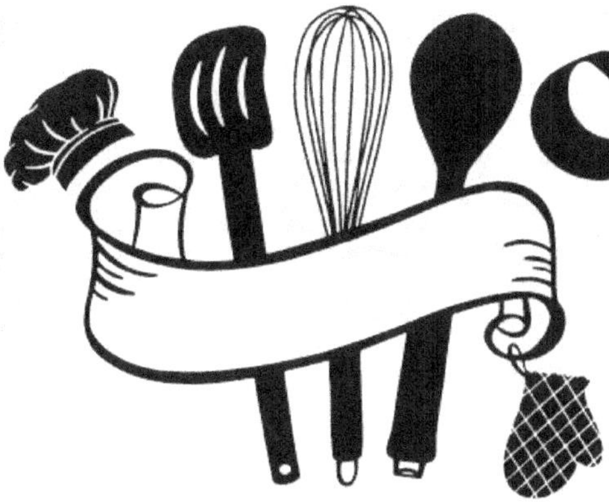

conversion chart

FOR THE KITCHEN

VOLUME MEASUREMENT CONVERSIONS

VOLUME MEASUREMENT CONVERSIONS

Cups	Tablespoons	Teaspoons	Milliliters
1/16 cup	1 tbsp	1 tsp	5ml
1/8 cup	2 tbsp	3 tsp	15 ml
1/4 cup	4 tbsp	6 tsp	30 ml
1/3 cup	5 1/3 tbsp	12 tsp	60 ml
1/2 cup	8 tbsp	16 tsp	80 ml
2/3 cup	10 2/3 tbsp	24 tsp	120 ml
3/4 cup	12 tbsp	32 tsp	160 ml
1 cup	16 tbsp	36 tsp	180 ml
		48 tsp	240 ml

1 QUART =
2 pints
4 cups
32 ounces
950 ml

1 PINT =
2 cups
16 ounces
480 ml

1 CUP =
16tbsp
8 ounces
240 ml

1/4 CUP =
4 tbsp
12 tsp
2 ounces
60 ml

1 TBSP =
3 tsp 1/2
ounce
15 ml

COOKING TEMPERATURE CONVERSIONS

Celcius/Centigrade $\qquad$ $F=(C \times 1.8) + 32$

Fahrenheit $\qquad$ $C=(F-32) \times 0.5556$

BAKING INGREDIENT CONVERSIONS

BUTTER

Cups	Grams
1/4 cup	57 grams
1/3 cup	76 grams
1/2 cup	113 grams
1 cup	227 grams

PACKED BROWN SUGAR

Cups	Grams	Ounces
1/4 cup	55 grams	1.9 oz
1/3 cup	73 grams	2.58 oz
1/2 cup	110 grams	3.88 oz
1 cup	220 grams	7.75 oz

ALL-PURPOSE FLOUR / CONFECTIONER'S SUGAR

Cups	Grams	Ounces
1/8 cup	16 grams	563 oz
1/4 cup	32 grams	1.13 oz
1/3 cup	43 grams	1.5 oz
1/2 cup	64 grams	2.25 oz
2/3 cup	85 grams	3 oz
3/4 cup	96 grams	3.38 oz
1 cup	128 grams	4.5 oz

GRANULATED SUGAR

Cups	Grams	Ounces
2 tbsp	25 grams	89 oz
1/4 cup	67 grams	1.78 oz
1/3 cup	50 grams	2.37 oz
1/2 cup	100 grams	3.55 oz
2/3 cup	134 grams	4.73 oz
3/4 cup	150 grams	5.3 oz
1 cup	201 grams	7.1 oz